overcoming weight problems

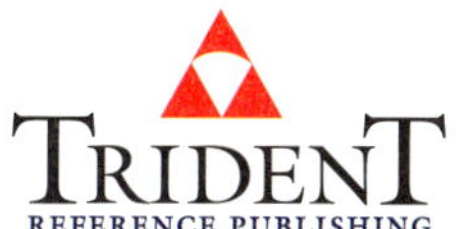

NOTE
This publication is intended to provide reference information for the reader on the covered subject. It is not intended to replace personalized medical diagnosis, counseling, and treatment from a doctor or other healthcare professional.
Before taking any form of treatment you should always consult your physician or medical practitioner.
The publisher and authors disclaim any liability, loss, injury or damage incurred as a consequence, directly or indirectly, of the use and application of the contents of this book.

Published by:
Trident Reference Publishing
801 12th Avenue South, Suite 400
Naples, Fl 34102 USA
Phone: + 1 239 649 7077
Email: sales@trident-international.com
Website: www.trident-international.com

Overcoming Weight Problems

Publisher
Simon St. John Bailey

Editor-in-chief
Isabel Toyos

Art Director
Aline Talavera

Photos
© Trident Reference Publishing,
© Getty Images, © Jupiter Images,
© Planstock, © J. Alonso

Includes index
ISBN 1582799717 (hc)
UPC 615269997178 (hc)
ISBN 1582799598 (pbk)
UPC 615269995983 (pbk)

2005 Edition
Printed in USA

overcoming weight problems

4 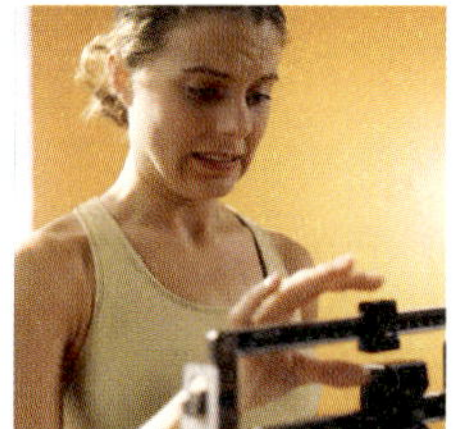 Introduction

20 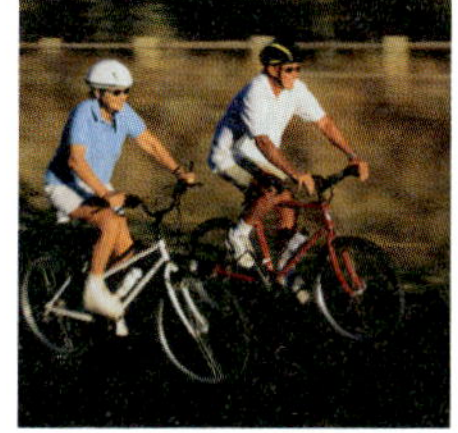 Diet and Weight Reducing Therapies

50 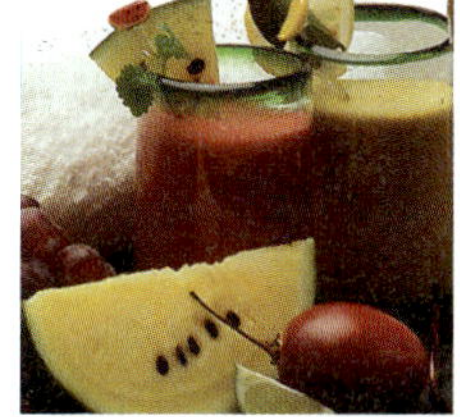 Healing Foods

56 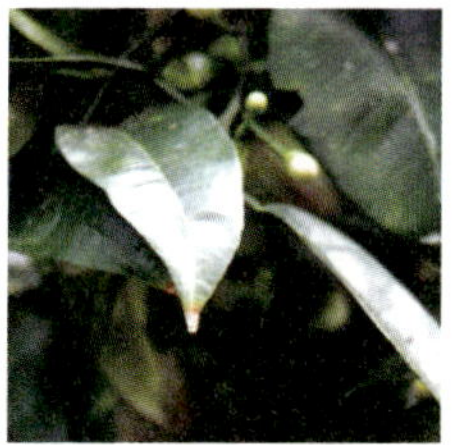 Natural Herb Remedies

What are weight problems?

Doctors usually define "overweight" as a condition in which a person's weight is 10 percent higher than "normal", as defined by a standard, height/weight chart, according to age, weight and physical type. Other than affecting our self-image, being overweight can have serious health consequences.

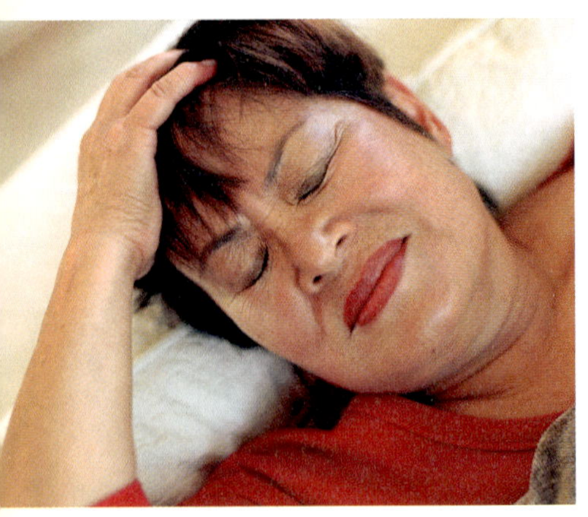

Overweight is defined as excess body weight, at the cost of an increase in fatty tissue, at no more than 10 percent higher than a healthy weight according to the age, height and body type of each individual.
In most cases the first indicators of weight gain are reflected in the way our bodies look and feel: when our clothes are tight and the way we look in the mirror, can be indicators of excess fat. We shouldn't ignore the first signs of weight gain, because overweight isn't only a problem of how we look, but also a sign of our state of health.

Most people think that gaining weight and getting older go hand in hand. Recent studies tell us that's just not true. If when you are 25 years old and have a normal, healthy weight range, over the years your weight should stay the same or go up no more than 11 lb/5 kg. Also, people often believe that it's "normal" that blood pressure increases with age, when studies have shown there are no physiological reasons for these changes. Studies have shown that excessive weight gain may be related to changes in blood pressure. This is just one example of the health problems brought on by being overweight.

OVERWEIGHT, OBESITY AND HEALTH

Controlling your weight and preventing obesity is the first step in reducing the risk of non-transmittable chronic diseases such as diabetes type II, high blood pressure, cardiovascular illnesses and some types of cancer, including of the uterus (in women) and of the prostate (in men). Excess weight can also have damaging effects on the skeleton. It can affect the joints, especially the knees, ankles, legs and back. These discomforts are generally painful and are accompanied by swelling and the bad posture that make physical activity more difficult. This causes a chain reaction of reduced mobility and therefore increased body weight.

In addition, there are a number of other health problems brought on by being overweight and carrying the risk of becoming obese: varicose veins, sleep apnea, fatty liver disease and dermatological problems caused by the fungus that grows in the folds of the flesh, where there is humidity. Overweight is also linked with uterine and postmenopausal breast cancer in women and prostate cancer in men. Gaining weight during adult life increases the risk of these cancers.
Weighing too much may put you at risk of developing many health problems. If you have a problem, you should visit your physician to see how you can lower your weight primarily to protect your health.

PEAR OR APPLE?

When we talk about "pear" or "apple" body shape, we are talking about where weight gain accumulates and the health risks related to body shape.

- **Apple.** People who tend to gain weight mostly in the waist area have more of an "apple" shape. Fatty tissue builds up around the waist and chest. If you are an "apple" rather than a "pear," you are at increased risk of the health problems associated with obesity, such as diabetes, coronary heart disease, and high blood pressure.

- **Pear.** "Pear-shaped" people carry their extra weight below the waistline, and do not seem to have as high a risk of developing the above conditions as "apples" do. However "pear shaped" figures have greater possibilities of suffering from leg, back and reverse blood flow circulation problems.

Most frequent causes

In most cases, people gain weight because they're eating more calories than they burn with physical activity. Without a doubt, sedentary lifestyle habits contribute to weight gain, but in most cases, people put on extra pounds/kilos despite an active lifestyle because they are not eating correctly.

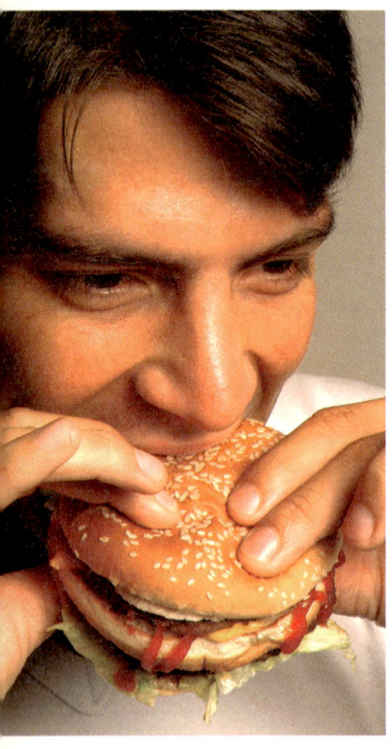

What are the major food mistakes that make us gain wait? We've included a list with the most important mistakes:

- If you eat large servings or have seconds.
- Adopting bad eating habits: eating high calorie foods or foods with low nutritional value but high in calories. For example, high-fat foods. Fat is a nutrient that has double the calories of carbohydrates and proteins. Butter, cream, mayonnaise, oil, lard, nuts, chocolate, cheese, fatty meat, deli meats and sausages are all foods high in calories and fat content. Fatty foods have another disadvantage, it's more difficult to control servings because they're sometimes more convenient and are very flavorful, making us crave them.
- Eating between meals without paying attention to what or how much you're eating. Snack foods tend to be high in calories and low in nutrients, playing a key factor in weight gain.
- Not eating enough fruits and vegetables.

They are high in fiber and water and low in fat and calories. At the same time they have a lot of volume and texture to fill you up. Fruits and vegetables need to be chewed well, making you eat slower.

To know if bad eating habits are the cause of your disgust with the weighing scales, answer the questions in the following quiz. It may help you to know if you are eating properly.

Results

Mostly answered A. Reflect, you are eating many foods high in fat. Think about solutions that my help you choose better eating habits.

Mostly answered B. Your habits are fairly healthy, you are probably less likely to have weight problems than other people.

ARE YOU EATING WELL? **A** **B**

1. What do you normally eat for breakfast?

A Picking up a quick cup of coffee and doughnut or pastry

B Before leaving the house, you have a breakfast with skimmed milk or yogurt, whole-grain bread, fruit and light cheese.

2. What do you do when you can't sleep?

A You get up to eat something to help you sleep.

B You get up and prepare a glass of warm milk. You take it to the bedroom and sip it slowly to help you get to sleep.

3. On the weekend....

A You sit on the couch watching television

B You go out for a walk or walk around the mall.

4. If you are overworked...

A You decide to not lose time in going out for lunch, you end up eating a quick sandwich, crackers and soda.

B You take 15 to 20 minutes to prepare a quick, light meal (instant soup, tomato, fruit or yogurt).

5. If you don't have anything at the house to cook for dinner...

A You call a restaurant for home delivery.

B You look for something in the pantry and decide on a can of tuna and fruit or make pasta.

6. If you meet a friend at a coffee shop, what do you order?

A Desert and coffee.

B A coffee or diet soda.

The ideal weight

It's not enough to weigh yourself or look in a mirror: there are exact formulas to indicate what is your appropriate weight according to your body type, sex and age.

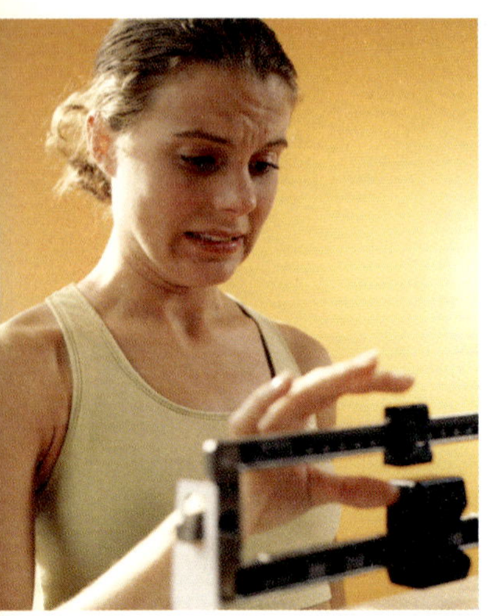

Generally, when you want to find out how much you weigh you simply get on the scales and find out if you've gone up or down a few pounds/kilos. Sometimes you're disappointed, sometimes enthused. However, your weight can be measured more precisely. Everyone has a different body type, and our weight does not always reflect if we are carrying extra pounds or if our body is healthy. There are a number of ways to precisely measure if our weight is healthy, using methods accepted by international health organizations.

The ways to measure:

■ **1. Body Mass Index.** Body Mass Index or BMI is now the most common tool used to measure obesity. To calculate your BMI the first step is stepping on a scale to find out how much is your real weight (without shoes and with light clothing). Next, find out your actual height, making sure to stand up straight. Stand with your head, buttocks, and feet touching a vertical wall. If this is not possible due to large amounts of body fat, simply stand erect; with hands relaxed at your sides. Look forward and keep your head straight and in an upright position. (You may be surprised because you thought your height was higher. Your height can vary with your age, if the vertebrae in the spine begin to compress. Bad posture, sedentary lifestyle and lack of stretching generally cause this). BMI measures your weight relative to your height. The ideal range is 18.5-24.9. A person with a BMI between 25 and 30 is considered to be overweight and a BMI over 30 indicates obesity (see *Are you overweight?* box).

■ **2. Measuring your waist.** Another way to find out if you are at risk of being overweight is by measuring your waist. You should measure your waist precisely (see *Your waist is your health* box). The WHO (World Health Organization) reports that a healthy person's waist should measure a maximum of 31.5 in/80 cm for women and 37 in/94 cm for men. If your waist measures more than these figures, it's a red light indicating that you are overweight. When the measurement is over 34.5 in/88 cm for women and 40 in/102 cm for men it's a sign that you are at serious risk, because there is an increase in fatty tissue around the digestive organs in the abdominal area, this type of weight gain can be very risky for the health.

■ **3. Body fat percentage.** This figure is obtained with the Deurenberg figure, which requires a number of calculations. Normally medical specialists or nutritionists can work out this figure. The result is a percentage that indicates whether you are overweight.

YOU WAIST IS YOUR HEALTH

The waist circumference is a reliable method of estimating the intra-abdominal fat mass and measuring your weight. To make sure you are taking the measurement properly keep in mind:

- *Don't measure the waist level you use for your clothes, but measure a little bit above the belly button.*
- *The recommended level is halfway between the iliac crest (the hipbone) and the edge of the last and lowest rib.*

ARE YOU OVERWEIGHT?

Find out how to calculate your BMI. To use this calculation you need to know your exact weight. The following is the formula:

$$\frac{\textbf{Weight}}{\textbf{Height}^2}$$

Depending on the results of the calculation, you'll know if your weight is healthy:

- **Underweight**: when the BMI is less than 18.5.
- **Normal or healthy weight**: when your BMI is between 18.6 and 24.9.
- **Overweight**: when the BMI is between 25 and 29.9.
- **Obesity**: when your BMI is more than 30.

Healthy habits

Eating well to keep our bodies healthy and strong doesn't mean only getting the necessary amount of essential nutrients, but also adopting healthy habits when eating meals.

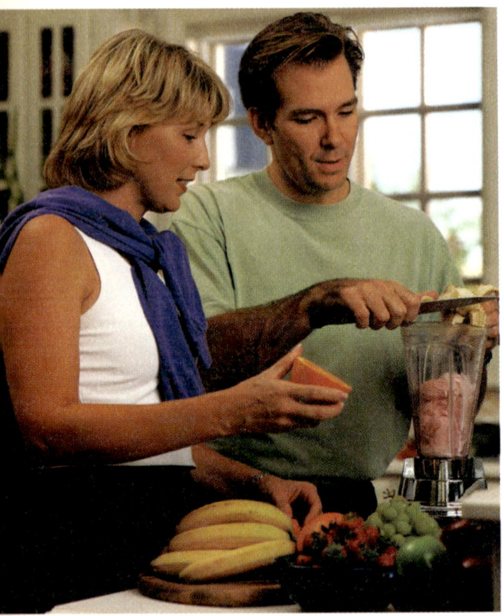

Eating properly doesn't imply only getting enough nutrients or eating in a disorderly manner. To make sure that foods are absorbed properly in the body for them to really be effective in supporting the health and keeping your weight under control you should make sure to:

Don't skip breakfast.

- This is the first meal after the fast of the night which has allowed your digestive

MAKE SURE TO EAT DURING BREAKFAST

To kick start your day with a healthy meal, your breakfast should include:

- **At least one low-fat, high-fiber energetic food: whole grain cereal, wholewheat bread, fruit.**
- **At least one low fat, high protein: skim dairy products such as milk, yogurt, or cream cheese.**
- **Quickly absorbed sugar (only when your weight is low): sugar, jams, and honey.**
- **Healthy fats (only when your weight is low): nuts.**
- **Plenty of liquids, in juices, water or infusions.**

EATING SAFE FOOD

When food isn't fresh make sure to:

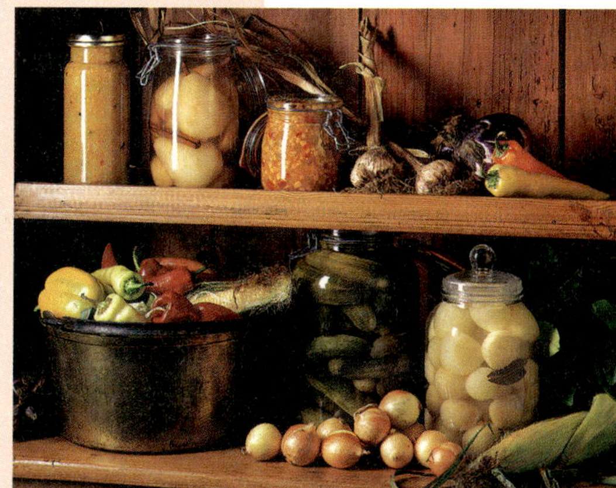

- **Don't eat foods that have been prepared in unsanitary conditions.**
- **Throw out any dented or pinched canned foods.**
- **Observe expiry dates.**
- **Don't refreeze foods and make sure foods stay chilled.**
- **Remember that although the freezer keeps food from developing bacteria, when you defrost it you should put it in the refrigerator or straight into the microwave immediately before cooking.**
- **Don't keep foods out of the refrigerator for very long.**
- **Make sure meat is cooked properly; only when the center reaches 158 °F/70 °C can you be sure that all bacteria have been destroyed by cooking.**
- **Carefully wash all fruit and vegetables.**

system to rest. Breakfast should keep the body energized and the mind clear all day long.

■ **Don't go long periods of time without eating during the day.** One of the main culprits of weight gain is not eating anything for prolonged periods, because you are distracted or busy. It modifies your metabolism and when you finally eat, hunger and anxiety make it difficult to control what foods you're eating and the size of servings. You are more likely to eat junk food or over eat, making you gain weight over time.

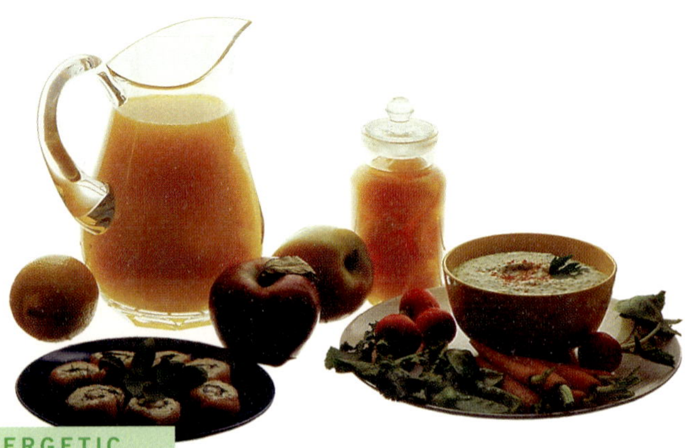

ENERGETIC LUNCH

A lunch in low fat proteins (fish, lean meats and egg whites) and complex carbohydrates from fruits and vegetables helps to keep your mind alert and calm, satisfying your appetite, because the meal incorporates all nutrients that you need. Carbohydrates for energy to help you work, aminoacids to improve neurotransmission and the break down and synthesis of proteins. Your body breaks down these nutrients slowly, providing energy for the whole day.

■ **Make sure that lunch serves its purpose.** That's to say that lunch provides you with the energy and nutrients that you need to help keep you going and keep you alert. Lunch shouldn't make you feel drowsy or sleepy because of the extra work breaking down food.

■ **Don't skip afternoon snack.**

- A long interval between lunch and dinner is the worst enemy of weight control.
- The path to weight gain is "picking" before meals. If you get home tired and hungry before dinner, you are more likely to pick at snack foods like cheese, deli meat, crackers and wine, that have more calories than a well-planned meal.

■ **Eat a well-balanced dinner.**

- To keep you healthy, you should keep in mind that dinner should provide you with the nutrients your body needs.
- The best dinner should complement your lunch.
- Remember that while lean proteins help

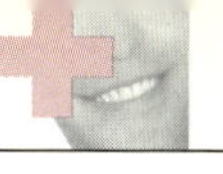

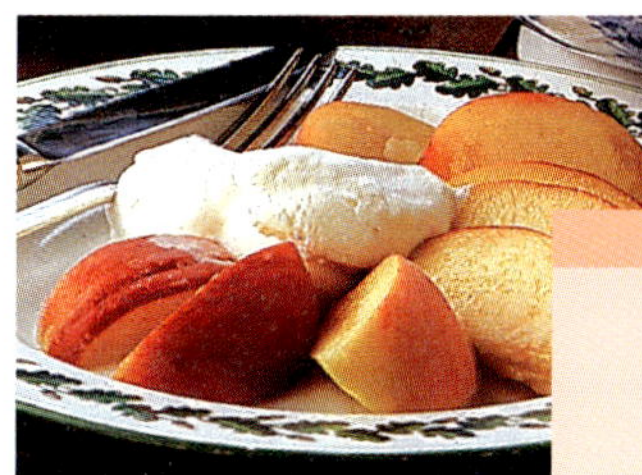

PERFECT COMBINATION

A combination of pasta, vegetables and a low-sugar dessert like yogurt or fruit, with milk or cheese is a great option for dinner.

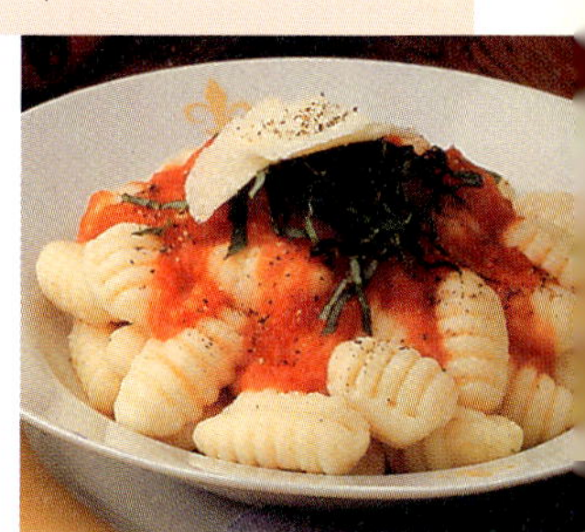

keep you alert, complex carbohydrates in pastas and grains and the sleep inducing aminoacid tryptophan in milk give off serenity and calm to help you get the repairing sleep you body needs.

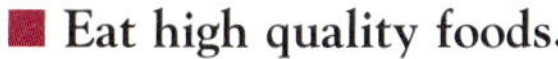

■ **Eat high quality foods.**

- It's important to look for and opt for foods that are low in fat, especially low in saturated fats.
- Stay away from trans fats. Carefully, look at nutrition labels to find out if the foods have hydrogenated oils added. We should get fats naturally from foods like lean meats and dairy products, which provide more than enough to stay healthy. Excess fats are harmful for the health.
- It's important to carefully read food labels on packaging to find out the nutritional information and ingredients.
- You should check to see how much fiber is found in food, and opt for products that have a higher amount of fiber per serving.
- You can also find out from food labels how much calcium and iron is found in the food product. Its best to choose foods that are low in fat and calories, but high in essential nutrients.

Quality in foods and eating

Eating isn't only about nutrition, it's also important to enjoy food with comfort and safety. Eating is a basic human need; sometimes we forget that food should be afforded more value than we tend to give.

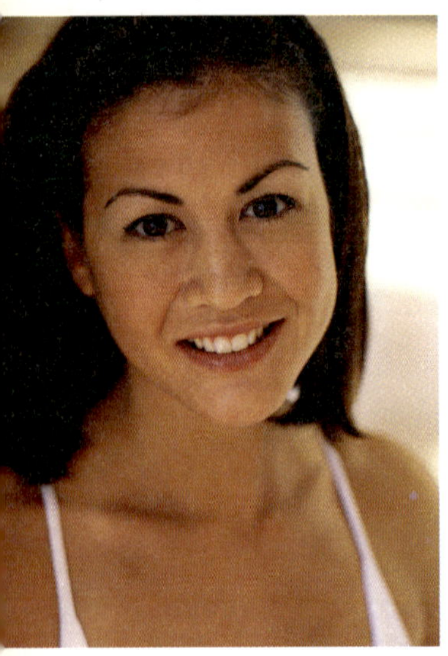

We eat many meals in our lifetime: approximately four times a day multiplied by every day of our lives. However, few times do we stop to reflect about the importance of eating natural and healthy foods valuing the act of eating more can improve our attitude to food in general.

- **The physical value of nutrients.** When we feel hungry, when we go a period of time without eating, and the body needs energy, is what causes us discomfort when we feel hungry.

- **The value of eating for pleasure.** Many times, the pleasure we get from foods is placed before nutritional value. Sometimes our body doesn't benefit from the food we eat. We develop, through culture and convenience, what pleasure we get for food. This is what makes us grab foods that are unhealthy to satisfy our appetites. We generally eat unhealthily because of convenience or because the food is rich in flavor, without keeping in mind that the food is high in carbohydrates (white flour, sugar) and fat. This is one of the paths to becoming overweight.

■ **Real nutritional value.** Nutritional value should be the first factor that we keep in mind when eating, although we don't always take this into consideration. What we learn from the ABC of what our bodies need to stay healthy we should use to plan meals accordingly, the body thanks you with a feeling of well-being. And remember, that eating healthily doesn't mean sacrificing flavor or pleasure (see *Time to cook* box).

■ **Emotional factor.** Studies have shown that we don't always eat when we are hungry: sometimes we look for comfort, pleasure, emotion, distraction and understanding in food. Sometimes use food to make us feel better, substituting food for emotional help. This is another path to weight gain.

■ **Safety value.** Fresh foods that are prepared correctly contribute to good health, but when foods are mishandled they can put our health at risk. Contaminated food can make us sick and even cause death through FTD (Food Transmittable Diseases) in the following cases: because they contain pathogenic bacteria, because toxins have grown making the food dangerous, even mortally.
Through mishandling food, it has been contaminated with a toxic substance.
In some cases contaminated foods can be noticed simply by the way they look, by the color, flavor and any unnatural aspect of the food. However, in many cases it's very difficult to know whether the food has been contaminated. This is why it's especially important to make sure that you choose high quality foods that have been handled properly (see *Eating safe food*, on page 11).

TIME TO COOK

The correct handling and cooking of foods keeps your family safe. Follow these guidelines to preserve the nutritional value of foods:

- Don't reheat leftovers, because it destroys nutrients.
- Don't cook with too much water, a lot of essential vitamins and minerals are left in the water.
- Don't cook with extremely hot temperatures because heat destroys vitamins and minerals.

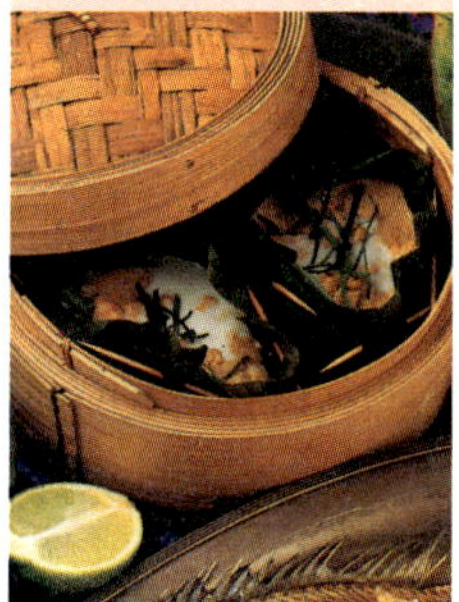

The role of the family

The family plays an important role in teaching healthy eating practices early on in life. It's important to teach children to approach eating with the right attitude.

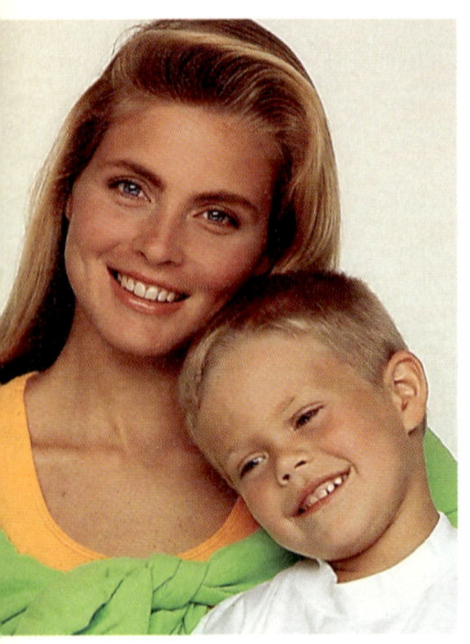

- Parents should try not to set children apart because of their weight, but focus on gradually changing their family's physical activity and eating habits. Family involvement helps to teach everyone healthful habits and does not single out the overweight child. Regular physical activity, combined with healthy eating habits, is the most efficient and healthful way to control your weight.
- Regular physical activity, combined with healthy eating habits, is the most efficient and healthful way to control your weight. Physical activity will help your child burn more calories.
- Limit the amount of "empty calories" (non-nutritious) foods, like highly sugared foods and regular soda.
- Decrease the amount of fat in daily meals and offer the whole family a wide variety of foods

SANDWICHES, GOOD OR BAD?

You should keep in mind that not all restaurant sandwiches are bad. Sandwiches can be practical and nutritious foods if they are prepared with wholewheat bread (with fiber), tomato slices and lean meat or hard cheese, but not as a daily option.

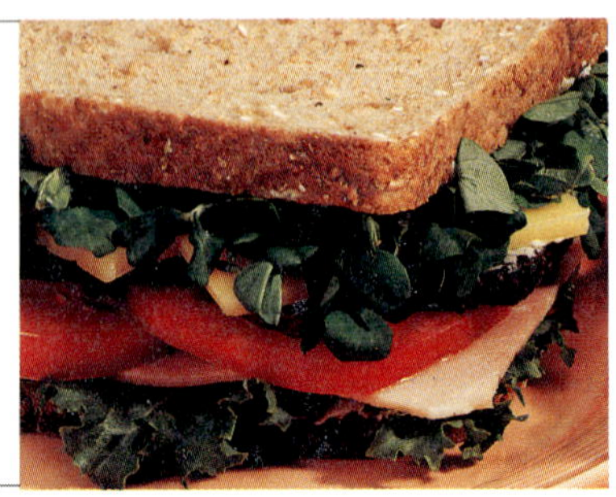

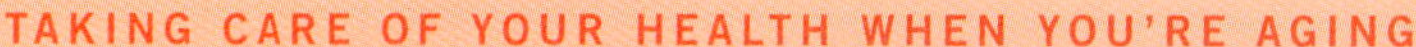

TAKING CARE OF YOUR HEALTH WHEN YOU'RE AGING

People who are elderly aren't destined to be overweight. Gaining weight is due to eating excessive amounts of refined foods and the lack of physical exercise. Some healthy habits you can incorporate during this stage of your life:

- Eating good proteins low in fat: skim milk (with fiber added), egg whites, fish and lean meat.
- The sugars found in fruit eaten daily provide a sufficient daily amount.
- Reduce the amount of salt in your foods and all foods that are processed with salt (deli meats and pre-packaged foods); this will help your cardiovascular health.
- If you want to get more calcium eat skim dairy products and whole grains.
- Vegetables should be included in every meal, because they support proper digestive function.
- If you don't eat meat, an egg is a good substitute.

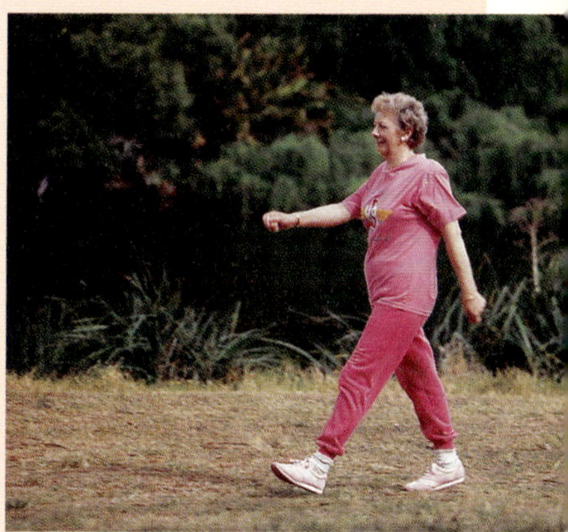

- You should increase the amount of foods rich in vitamin C (orange or lemon juice), that help in the absorption of iron from deep green leafy vegetables.
- You should increase your physical activity, with your family or on your own.

from each of the food groups, low in fat but rich in nutrients.

■ Control the amount of pre-packaged and processed foods.

■ Recreate traditional family recipes with a healthier version, using less vegetable oils and skim products, and whenever possible, avoiding sugars, sweets or honey.

■ Plan family activities that provide everyone with exercise and enjoyment like walking, dancing, biking, or swimming. Afterward, but not immediately afterward you can drink a mineral beverage. A piece of fruit, cereal bar or low-fat yogurt are some options for a healthy snack.

■ Reduce the amount of time you and your family spend in sedentary activities, such as watching TV, playing video games or in front of the computer.

Overweight children

More and more children and teenagers are overweight. Bad eating habits, lack of physical activity and sitting in front of the television and computer for hours are the principle causes. It's important to take immediate steps in improving your child's weight by gradually changing your family's physical activity and eating habits.

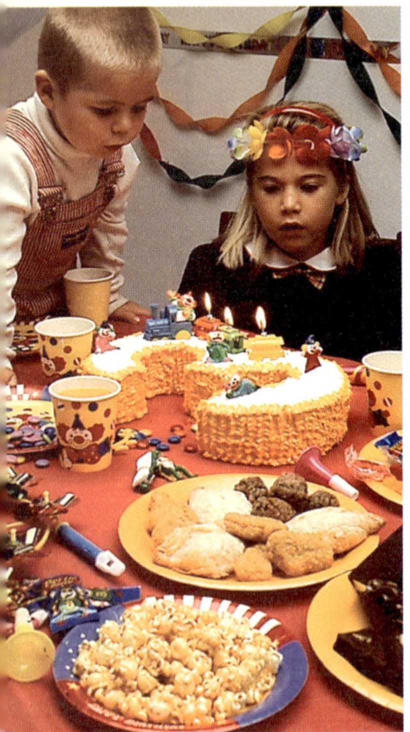

The percentage of children and teenagers who are overweight is alarming: over the last two decades, this number has increased by more than 50 percent, and the number of "extremely" overweight children has nearly doubled.

Children whose parents, brothers or sisters are overweight may be at an increased risk of becoming overweight themselves. Genetic factors play a role in increasing the likelihood that a child will be overweight. If a child has a mother or father who is obese there's a 40 percent chance he will also be obese. If both parents are obese, the percentage goes up to 80 percent. Although weight problems run in families, not all children with a family history of obesity will be overweight; shared family behaviors such as eating and exercise habits also influence body weight. Eating habits are generally developed during childhood, if a child's parents are obese they are likely to adopt unhealthy eating habits.

THE PLEASURE OF EATING AT HOME

Associating food with how we feel is one of the most common emotional mechanisms we learn in childhood. Children are taught daily that soda drinks are to celebrate and vegetables are a punishment, a type of necessary torture. Foods that are given to children as a type of prize or payment are going to turn into their favorite foods. While foods that they are forced to eat, will be progressively rejected. This is why it's important to teach children the pleasure in simple homemade foods, that have all the necessary nutrients for their growth.

Some parents think that the answer is to put their child on a strict diet, but this is not the long-term solution. The best way to begin is to learn more about children's nutritional needs by reading or talking with a health professional and then to offer your children some healthy options, allowing them to choose what and how much they eat. The practitioner will probably offer three strategies:

- Reducing the amount of fat in your child's diet.
- Increasing the amount of physical activity for your child.
- Identifying and treating your own habits about weight control.

In relation to the last point, it's important to watch your child's behavior to determine if he eats when he is anxious, bored or nervous. In these cases, parents should consult a therapist to accompany medical treatment.

Being overweight isn't only a physical condition; it is related to overall well-being.

SELF-ESTEEM

Obesity in children can cause problems for kids in relation to their self-image. They suffer from this problem because their classmates may poke fun at them, affecting their self-esteem. Once this attitude has been incorporated, it's difficult to reverse it. In general, kids who are overweight during adolescence and suffer from discrimination by their friends, family and school peer groups, tend to have problems in their adult lives.

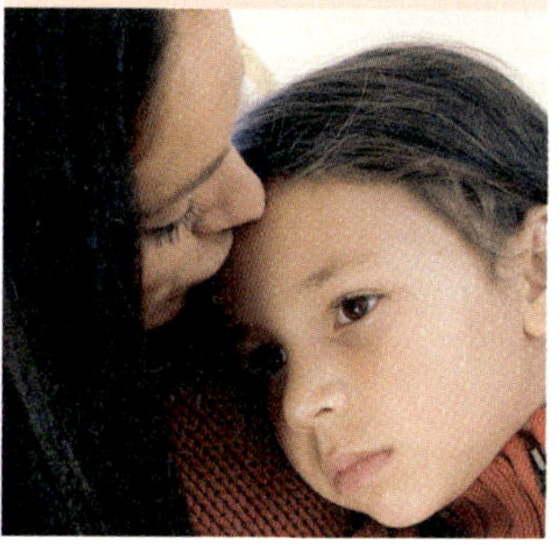

Design your own diet

When you know what healthy eating habits are, you can design a personalized diet to help lose weight, according to your particular needs. You only need to follow two basic rules: follow the food pyramid guidelines and cut down on serving sizes.

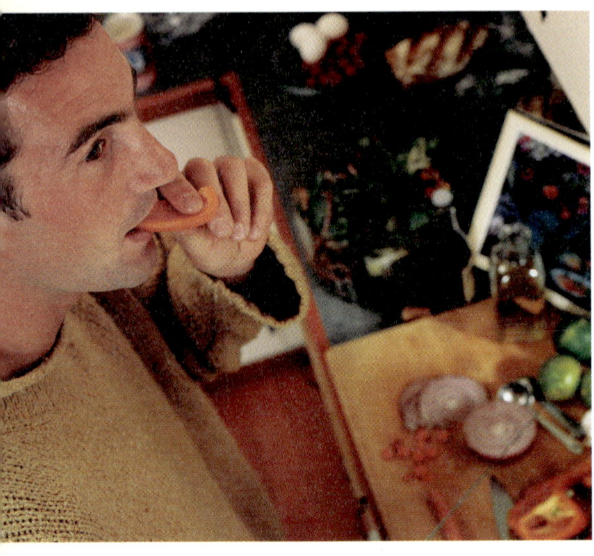

When planning a healthy diet to lose weight you should make sure that you choose foods from at least the five basic food groups. The groups for basic nutritional needs are:

- **Starches and grains.** Cereals and derivatives. Try to incorporate wholegrains (bread, pastas and flour). Other starches include root vegetables, starchy vegetables and beans.
- **Fruits and vegetables.** All types, of every color.
- **Proteins.** Animal products such as lean meats (red, poultry, fish and shellfish) and eggs. Tofu and soy is a vegetarian option.
- **Dairy products.** Milk, yogurt, cheeses, always choosing skim or hard cheeses.
- **Oils.** Vegetable oils, beans, avocados and seeds are the healthiest. Other less-healthy fats include butter, mayonnaise, cream and others.

STEP BY STEP DIET

To design a proper diet you shouldn't just keep in mind how many servings you should eat for proper nutrition, but also what does "a serving" mean. This will help you avoid making the mistake of overeating.

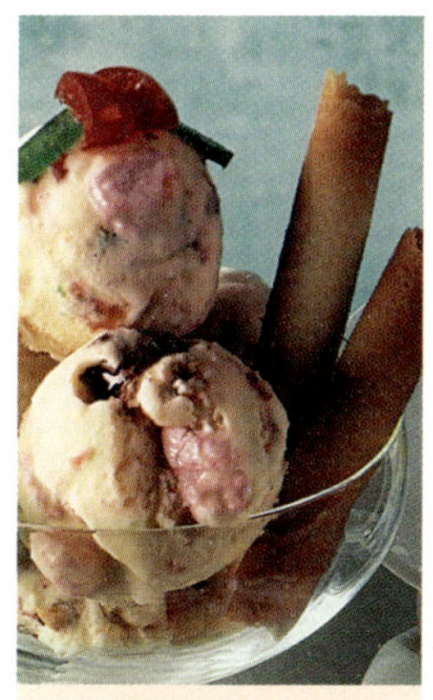

WARNING
While people with normal weight can eat sugar and consume alcohol in moderation, if you need to lose weight you should eliminate them from your diet altogether.

FIRST STEP
Knowing what and how much to eat

■ **Grains.** Recommended amount of grains is 5 equivalent servings to keep your weight under control. To lose weight, no more than 3 to 4 daily servings.

■ **Fruits and vegetables.** To keep your weight under control eat a minimum of 5 servings daily. If you are trying to lose weight eat 4 servings of vegetables and 3 fruit servings daily.

■ **Meat and eggs.** To stay healthy and to keep your weight under control 1 to 1 1/2 servings daily (making sure that you choose lean meat) is enough. To lose weight you need the same amount: 1 to 1 1/2 servings, but taking extreme care to eat only lean meats.

■ **Dairy products.** To stay healthy and keep your weight under control you need 3 servings daily (1 should be cheese), preferably natural hard cheese. To lose weight you need the same amount, but you should eat skim milk or yogurt and include one hard, natural cheese in this food group.

■ **Oils.** To stay healthy and keep your weight under control 2 to 4 servings are recommended, while prioritizing "good" fats (vegetable unsaturated). To lose weight you should include only 2 servings of "good" fats in your daily diet, use oils sparingly.

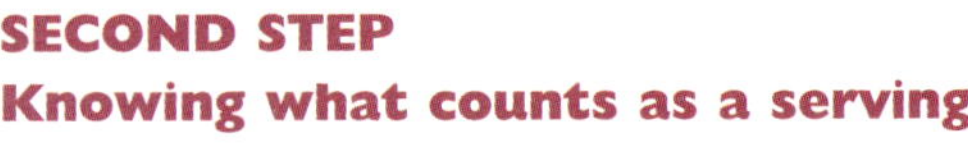

SECOND STEP
Knowing what counts as a serving

Before designing your daily diet, you should have on hand a list of the quantities for each group, that's to say how much is a serving for each food group and equivalent values. This information will help you design an appropriate diet according to your personal tastes, alternating a diverse range of foods for variety to help you stick with your healthy diet.

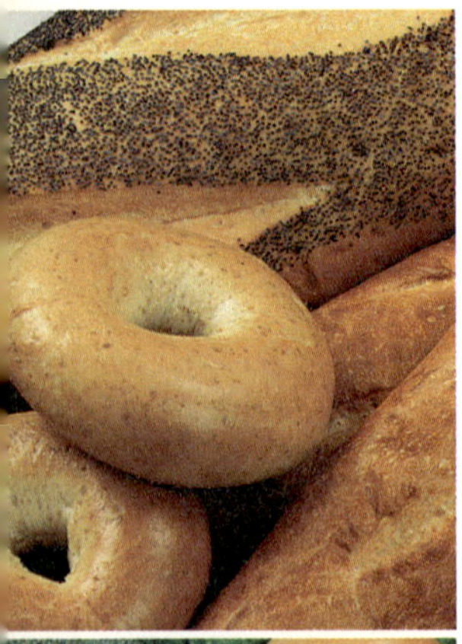

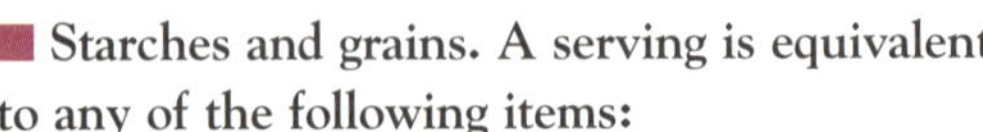

■ **Starches and grains. A serving is equivalent to any of the following items:**

- 1 small potato or sweet potato;
- 2-3 fine slices of potato, sweet potato or corn;
- 1 cup of cooked pasta;
- 1 cup of cooked grains (rice, millet, barley, wheat, oatmeal and other whole grains);
- 1 cup of cooked beans (white beans, lentils, chick peas, pinto beans and others;
- 1 small bun or pita bread;
- 2 slices of bread (best if it's wholewheat);
- 4 thin slices of French bread, toasted;
- 2 vanilla fingers or 2 Bay Biscuits;
- 20 oat cakes;
- 1/2 cup of breakfast cereal without sugar, preferably whole grain with fiber.

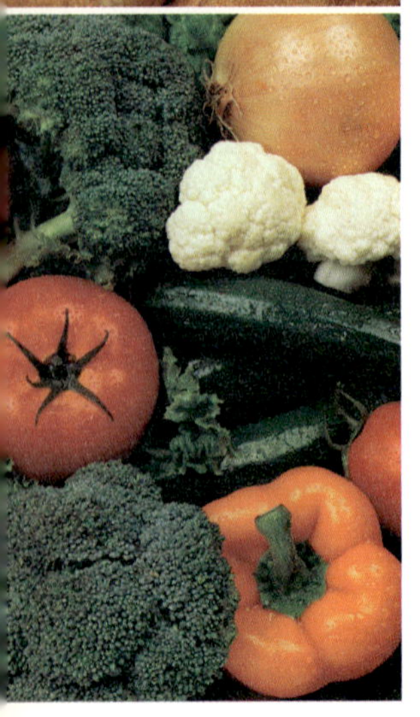

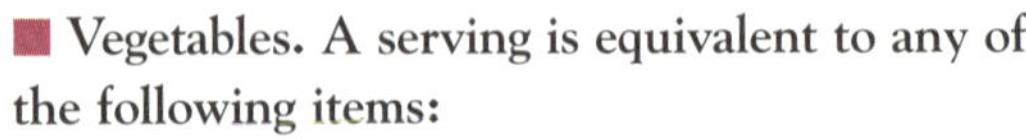

■ **Vegetables. A serving is equivalent to any of the following items:**

- 1 medium vegetable;
- 1 plate of various raw vegetables;
- 1 plate of cooked vegetables, not compressed;
- 2 slices of pumpkin;
- 1 cup of cooked vegetables, compressed.

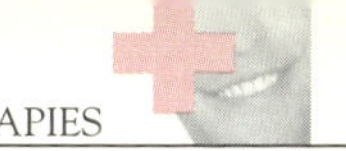

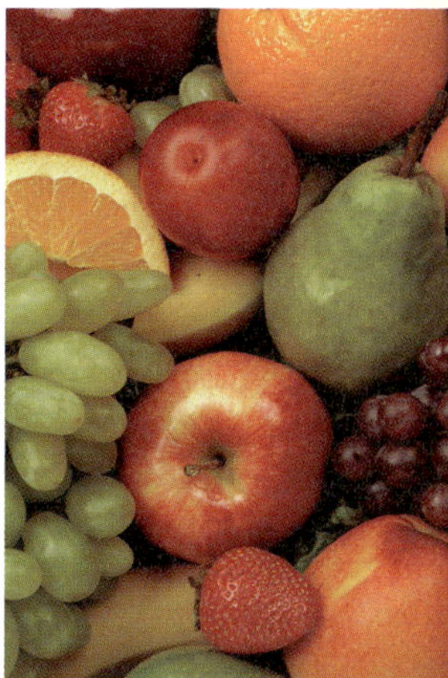

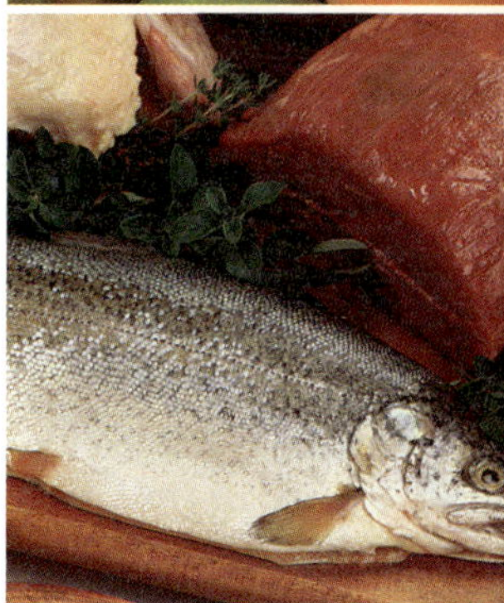

Fruit. A serving is equivalent to any of the following items:

- 1 small fruit (any fruit except banana);
- 1 cup of sliced fruit/strawberries/melon;
- 1/2 large fruit;
- 2 halves of canned fruit, sugar free;
- 1/2 small banana.

Meat-eggs and other proteins. A serving is equivalent to any of the following items:

- 1 small lean beef steak (4 in/10 cm in diameter);
- 2 thin slices of lean beef, roasted;
- 1 breaded thin steak; baked not fried;
- 1/4 small chicken, skinless, not fried;
- 1 small boneless chicken breast (or 1/2 medium), not fried.
- 1 small can of tuna in spring water, drained;
- 1 medium fish fillet;
- 1 fish steak;
- 1 egg or 2 egg whites;
- 3-4 thin slices of cured ham, very dry;
- 1 cup of tofu;
- 1 soy patty or soyburger.

Milk. A serving is equivalent to any of the following items:

- 1 glass of skim milk or yogurt (6 1/2 fl oz/ 200 cc);
- 3 tablespoons light cream cheese or skim ricotta cheese;
- 1 slice of natural, hard cheese (2 oz/60 g);
- 1 small slice of mozzarella cheese or semi hard cheese (1 oz/30 g);
- 2 thin slices of American cheese on a sandwich;
- 2 tablespoons of grated Parmesan cheese.

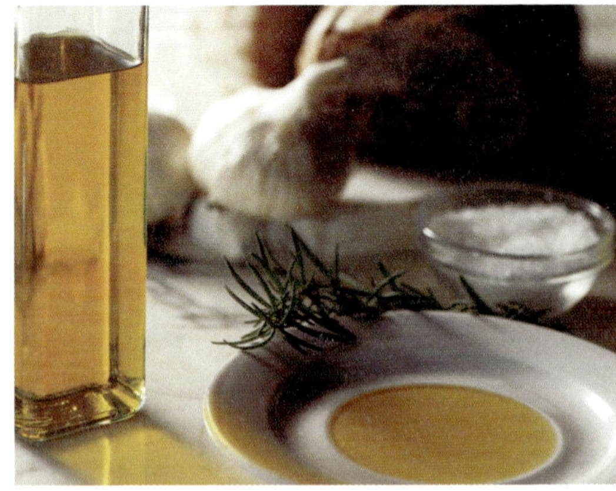

IMPORTANT
Always keep in mind that a serving is equivalent to the following: 1 cup = 6 1/2 oz/200 cc; 1 tablespoon = 1/2 oz/20 cc.

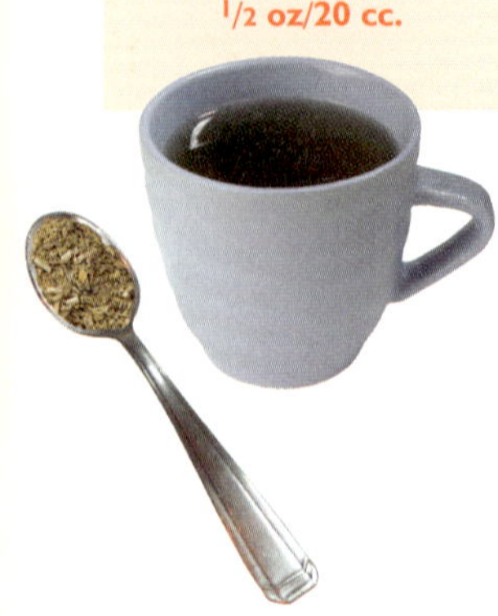

- **Oils. A serving is equivalent to any of the following items:**

Healthy fats

- 1 tablespoon of oil (best if it's olive or corn oil);
- 1 tablespoon of mayonnaise;
- 2 tablespoons of light mayonnaise;
- 4 tablespoons of avocado purée;
- 3 tablespoons of seeds or dry nuts.

Less healthy fats

- 1 tablespoon of butter or margarine;
- 2 tablespoons of light margarine;
- 3 tablespoons of light cream.

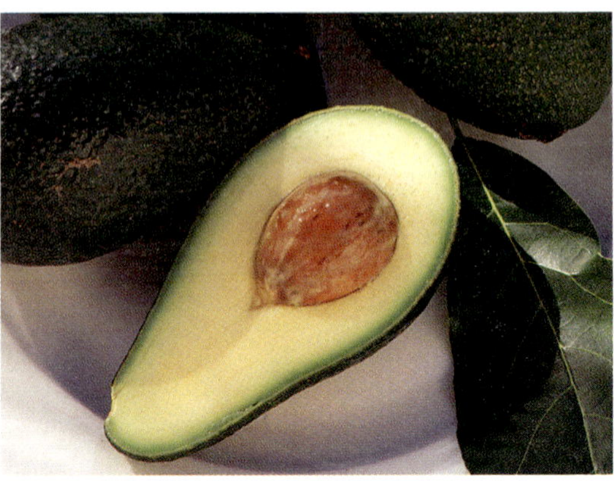

THIRD STEP
Designing your daily menu

Once you know the servings for each food type, you can design your own diet plan according to your own tastes and preferences. Just choose a serving of each food for each meal

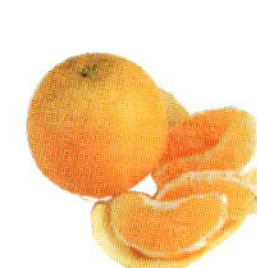

Breakfast

- 1 serving of fruit.
- 1 serving of grains.
- $1^1/_2$ servings of dairy products.
- Water.
- 1 infusion without sugar.

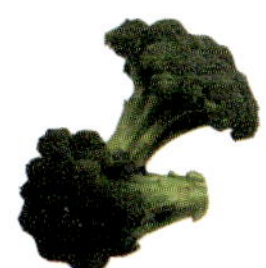

Lunch

- 1 serving of raw vegetables.
- 1 serving of meat.
- 1 serving of cooked vegetables.
- 1 serving of oils.
- 1 serving of fruit.

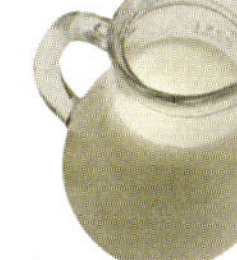

Snack

- $1^1/_2$ servings of dairy products.
- 1 serving of grains/starch.
- Water or calorie free drinks.
- 1 infusion without sugar.

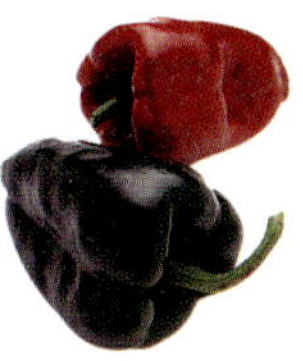

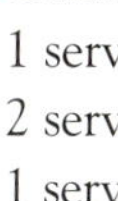

Dinner

- 1 serving of raw vegetables.
- 2 servings of grains.
- 1 serving of cooked vegetables.
- 1 serving of oils.
- 1 serving of fruit.

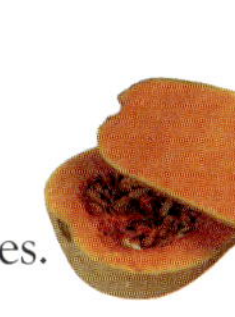

HEALTHY COOKING

To make sure that you're cooking healthily follow these easy steps:

- Brown vegetables in a nonstick pan, with a vegetable spray.
- Grill lean beef on a grill or broiler.
- Add lemon juice, water and a few drops of oil mixed together.
- Always steam, sauté or bake vegetables.
- Use sugar-free sweeteners. If you are baking, remember to use artificial sweeteners that tolerate heat.

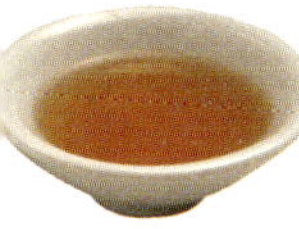

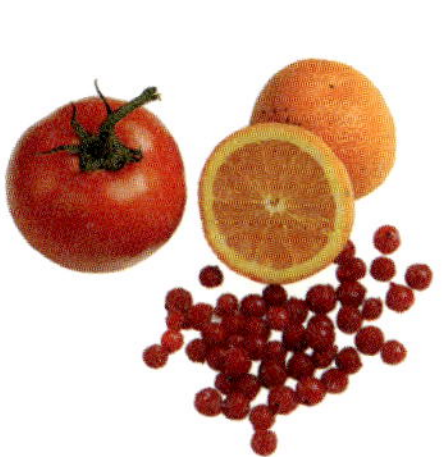

A model plan

The following diet plan is a model that you can use daily if you are thinking about gradually losing weight. Eat healthily and stick to serving sizes.

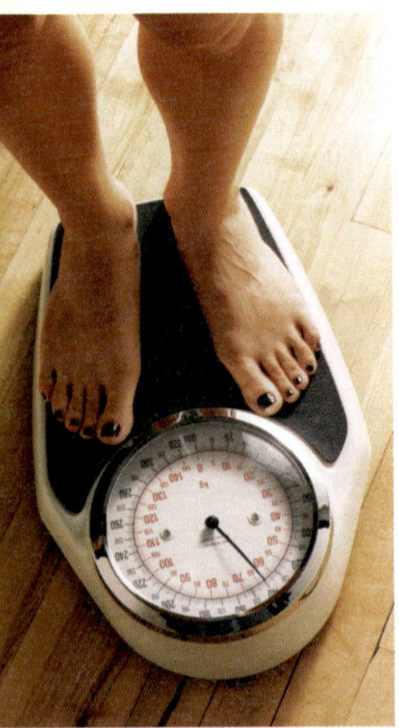

Breakfast

- 1 infusion.
- 1 glass of skim milk.
- 2 slices of wholewheat toast.
- 1 slice of sandwich cheese.
- 1 small orange.

Lunch

- Optional: a cup of vegetable broth.
- 1 plate of salad with tomato and leafy green lettuce.
- 2-3 thin slices of baked beef, with 1/2 pepper and 1/2 onion (1 serving of vegetables).
- 1 tablespoon of oil as a dressing.
- 2 plums.

Snack

- 1 cup of skim yogurt.
- 1 serving of pita bread.
- 1 slice of American cheese.
- 2 slices of tomato.
- Infusion or calorie free drink.

Dinner

- Grated carrot salad (with lemon).
- Rice with mushrooms and leeks (2 cups of cooked rice and 1 serving vegetable).
- 1 tablespoon of oil to cook the rice.
- 1 cup of fruit salad without sugar.

FOOD PYRAMID

- *The best way to make sure you are getting a complete and balanced diet, without complicated calculations of calories, cholesterol or fats, is by following the proportions indicated in what is called "the food pyramid" guide. Nutritionists agree that this graphic gives an overview of what is considered a complete, balanced diet.*
- *At the base of the pyramid are grains, which should make up the principle energy source for the body, fruits and vegetables, rich in vitamins and minerals. These foods are also rich in fiber, which aid in digestion.*
- *In the center are all the protein-based foods, important for the body but which can be harmful if eaten in excess.*
- *At the very top of the food pyramid appear fats and sweets, which are also necessary elements but should be limited and eaten in moderation.*
- *Current models of the food pyramid include references to physical exercise and drinking water, two direct factors in a balanced diet for a healthy weight.*
- *It's important to exercise at least 3 times a week and drink at least 8 glasses of water per day.*

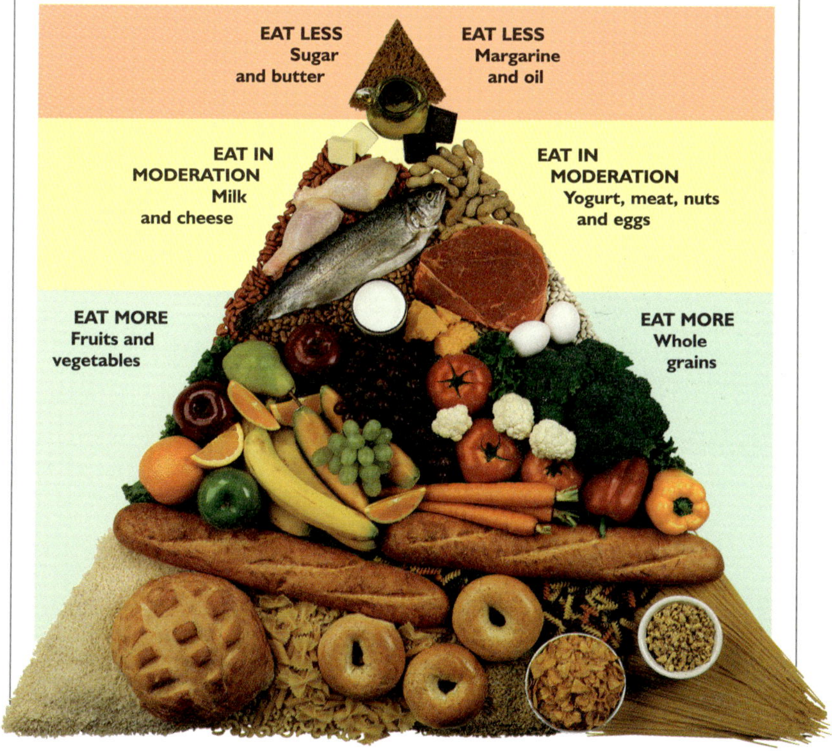

EAT LESS
Sugar and butter

EAT LESS
Margarine and oil

EAT IN MODERATION
Milk and cheese

EAT IN MODERATION
Yogurt, meat, nuts and eggs

EAT MORE
Fruits and vegetables

EAT MORE
Whole grains

Importance of moving

Avoiding a sedentary lifestyle is vital for good health. All physical activity practiced during the day is important for keeping your body in good physical shape.

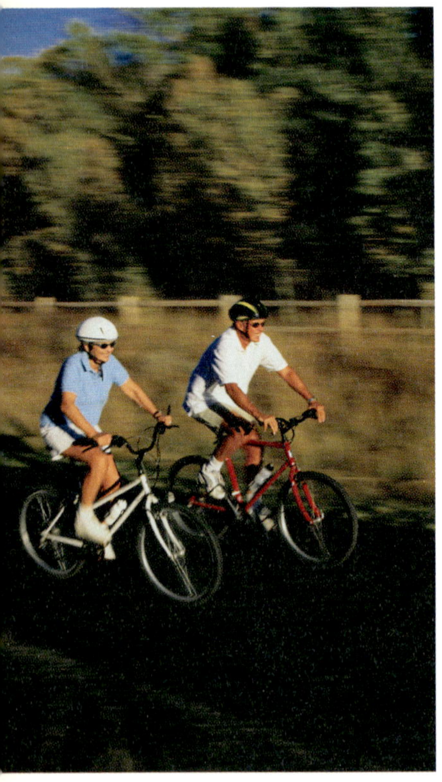

Exercise is especially recommended for people who are overweight. People who aren't used to a regular exercise routine can start by adding more physical activity in their daily routines. Exercising regularly implies that you are burning more calories, which is an important step along the path to weight loss. There are many simple and great ways to take advantage of your daily activity to include more exercises, build muscle mass and burn more calories. For example:

- In the mornings, wake up 15 minutes earlier and take a few minutes to stretch out your muscles.
- Use a stationary bicycle while watching TV.
- Whenever possible, walk up the stairs instead of taking the elevator. Even if you have to go up to the tenth floor, its best to take the elevator up to the ninth floor and then walk up the stairs to the tenth floor.

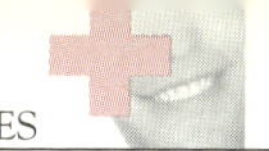

As your body builds up stamina, you can add a floor per week.

• Walk for 10 minutes three times a day: when shopping, taking the dog for a walk or going for a stroll. Another strategy is to take public transport get off one stop before your usual stop, and walk the few blocks to your location.

• Listen to music… and dance!

MORE VIGOROUS EXERCISES

Once you've got out of your sedentary habits and feel more energetic, you can slowly increase your activity and even join a gym. Try to briskly walk on a tread mill, go jogging, bike, go to the gym or start up a sport in which you burn calories. The important tip to remember is to stick with the exercise.

IS MY BODY READY?

Before beginning any exercise program it's important to visit your doctor to make sure that you don't have any health problems which exercising could complicate, or a particular exercise that

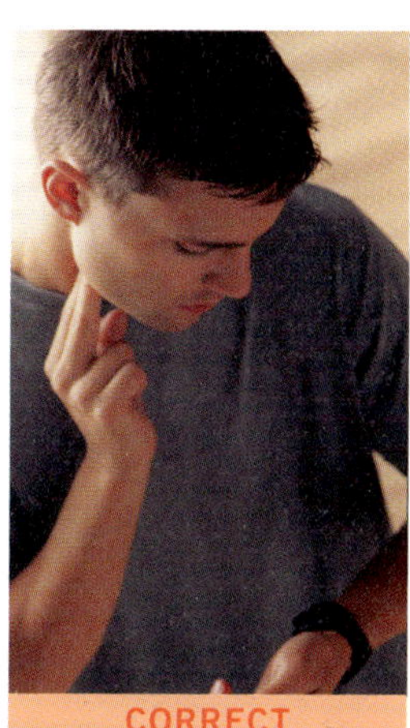

CORRECT EXERCISE

You shouldn't choose a physical activity based on the amount of calories that you burn during the exercise, but an activity that is fun for you and that you can fit into your daily routine. Whatever activity you choose you should begin with moderation, and slowly increase the intensity.

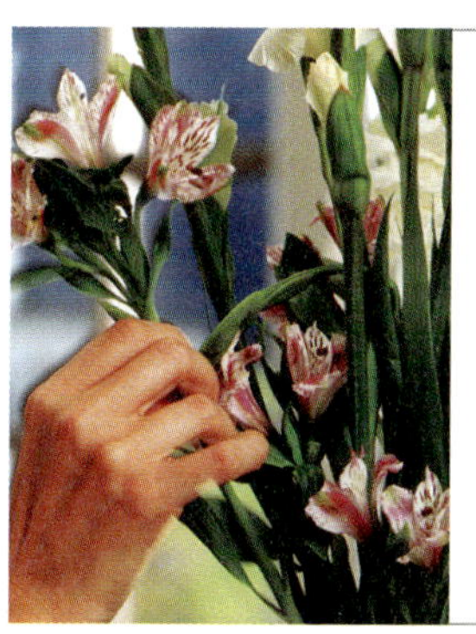

DAILY ACTIVITY AND CALORIES

Physical activity	Calories burned in 30 minutes
Sitting	40
Gardening or yard work	115
Cutting the grass	125
Washing windows	130
Vacuuming	130
Cleaning the floor	130
Sweeping	170

you shouldn't do. It's important if you suffer from any pain after exercising to visit your doctor for a professional medical opinion of what exercise is right for you. Keep in mind that some exercises or sports can be challenging for some but very beneficial for others.

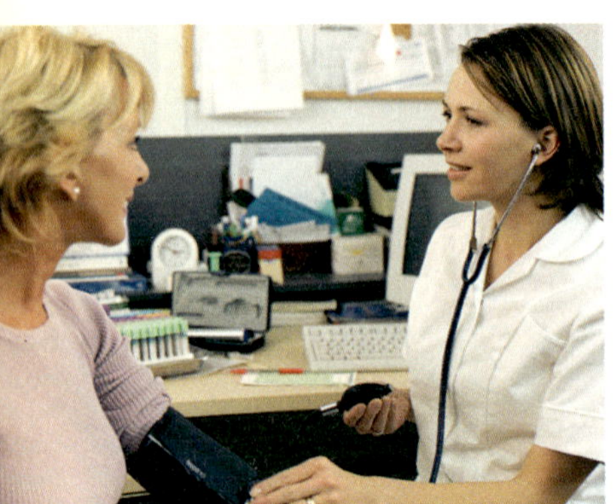

Once you've visited your doctor, it's important that you choose an exercise that you like and have fun. This is important so that you continue with your exercise program. To reaffirm your commitment to improving your health, it may help to write it down. For example:

My goal is to practice (write the exercise you've chosen)..

for (write the amount)...............................

minutes per day, (write the amount)................

times a week.

ACTIVE KIDS

We all know that it's more comfortable for parents to give their kids a lift to school or pick them up, or for their kids to take the bus. But it's ideal for kids to walk to school and back home (if you accompany them, you're also getting exercise!).

This is one of the best and most unforced ways of motivating them to exercise when

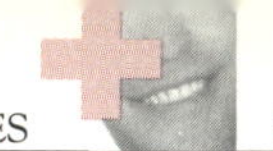

CALORIES BURNED WITH MODERATE PHYSICAL EXERCISE

Physical exercise	Calories burned in 30 minutes
Biking (5miles/8 km per hour)	*105*
Walking (2.5 miles/4 km per hour)	*105*
Low impact aerobic	*120*
Rowing	*130*
Golf	*150*
Swimming	*150*
Water aerobics	*175*
Volleyball	*175*

CALORIES BURNED WITH INTENSE PHYSICAL EXERCISE

Physical exercise	Calories burned in 30 minutes
Biking (10 miles/16 km per hour)	*195*
Skating (10 miles/16 km per hour)	*200*
Walking (4 miles/6.5 km per hour)	*220*
Tennis (singles)	*232*
Basket ball	*275*
Soccer	*350*
Weights	*378*
Taekwondo	*390*

they are young. Be a role model for your children. If your children see that you are physically active and having fun, they are more likely to be active and stay active for the rest of their lives. Reduce the amount of time you and your family spend in sedentary activities, such as watching TV or playing video games. For example, schedule a walk with your family after dinner instead of watching TV. Make sure that you plan activities that can be done in a safe environment.

THE BENEFITS OF PHYSICAL EXERCISE

Physical exercise helps to get rid of excess appetite and lose weight, but it also helps to:

- Get over states of tiredness and boredom.
- Deal with stress.
- Increase your energy.
- Reduce the risk of high blood pressure and diabetes.
- Lower cholesterol levels in the blood.

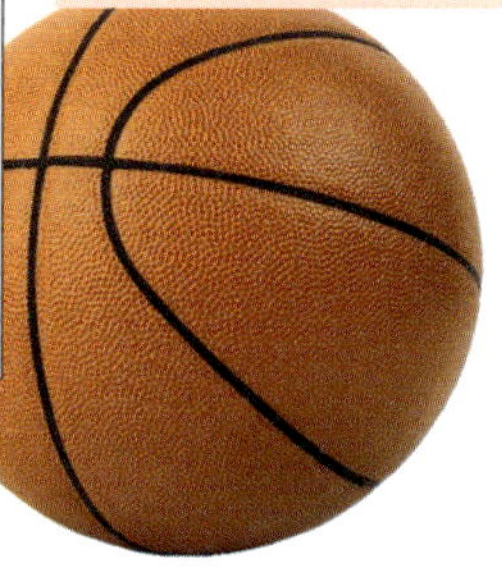

Walking for your health

Walking is the most natural physical activity, appropriate for people of all ages. Also, studies have proven that briskly walking works out the body as much as running or high-impact aerobics, but without putting your joints at risk.

IDEAL SHOE

You should be very careful in choosing your sports shoe. It should be flexible and comfortable with a cushioned and soft tongue, heel and toe. It should also support the foot. The heel should be slightly raised.

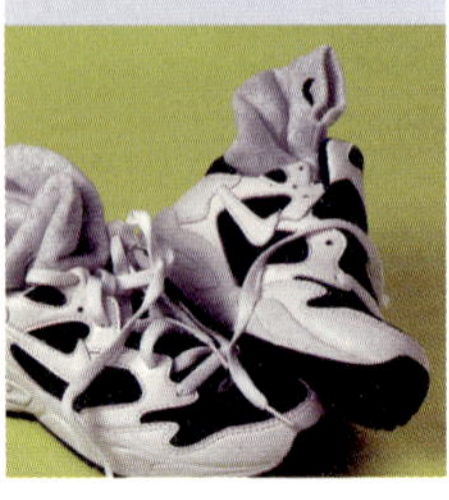

✚ To get the most out of walking as a workout you should pay attention to your posture, clothing and rhythm.

■ You should wear light clothing, preferably of cotton fiber (because it absorbs sweat). It's fundamental to wear comfortable shoes that support the feet without compressing them.

■ To avoid injuries, like falls or twisting your ankle, you should first warm up. Walk slowly for five minutes before picking up rhythm.

■ You should use a constant rhythm, until the last few meters of your walk, when you should use a slower rhythm.

■ If, when on your walk, you have up hill or down hill, you should go and return on the same route to make up for your effort either way.

■ Do 3 to 5 minutes of stretching before and after exercising. Stretch your arms, waist and legs to prevent any later pain or soreness from overstraining your muscles (see *Pre-workout stretch* box, on page 35).

SPORTS WALKING PROGRAM

When you choose walking as your work out activity you need to plan how much and how fast you are going to walk, keeping in mind

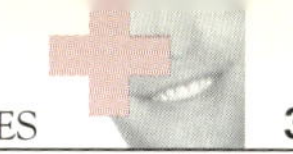

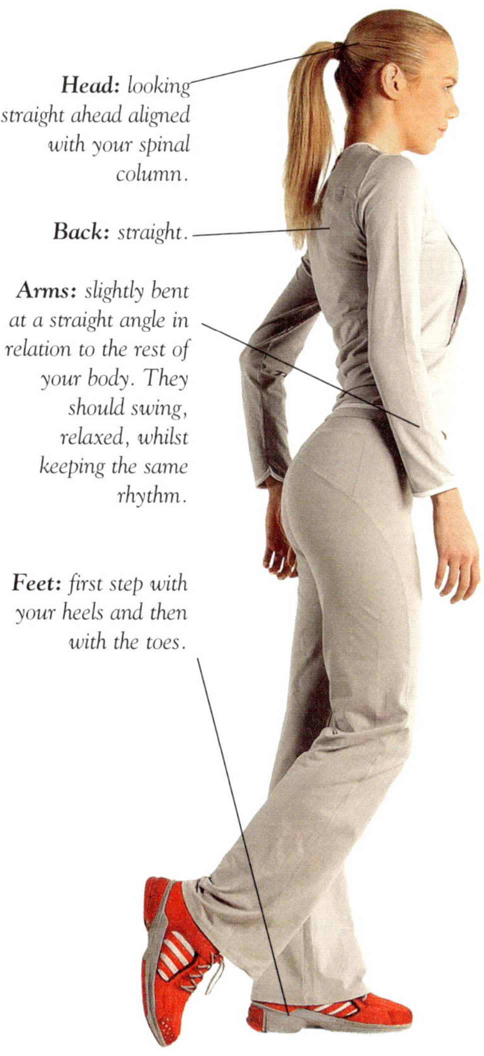

AEROBIC ACTIVITY

High intensity walking, as with all aerobic activity, causes an increase in your heart beat (amount of heartbeats per minute). The ideal frequency for this type of activity is 70% of: 220 minus the age of the person. For example, for a 40-year-old man it would be:

220 – 40 = 180

70% of 180 = 126

This means that for this man, his ideal heart rate during aerobic activity is 126.

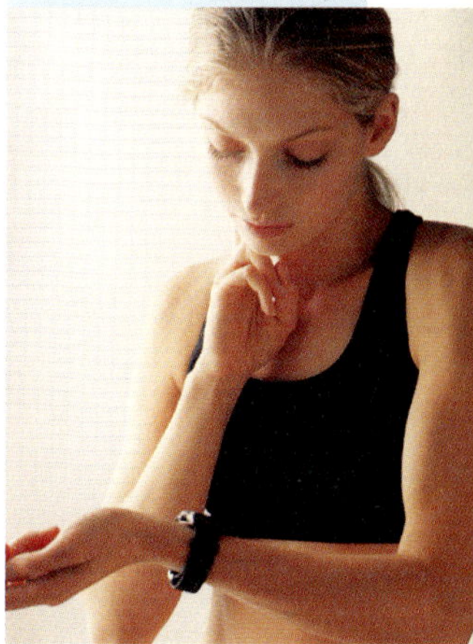

your physical shape and necessary training. We recommend starting with a moderate weekly routine, increasing the intensity as your body gains stamina and strength.

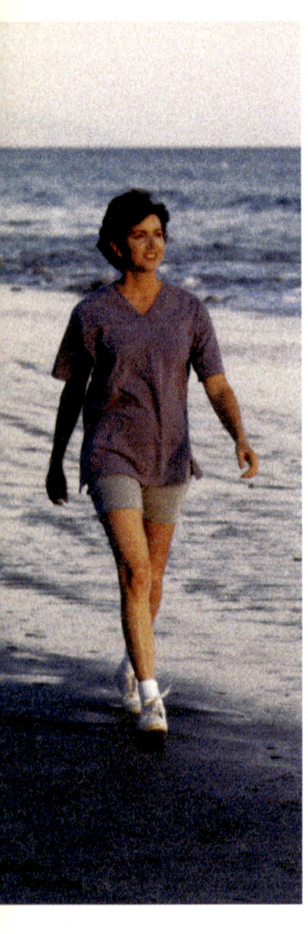

Walking for beginners

For obese people, sedentary or elderly, it's recommended that you begin by walking 10 blocks (1,100 yards/1,000 meters) in 12 to 15 minutes, 3 times a week. Increase the distance by 2 blocks per day, until you end up walking a total distance of 30 to 50 blocks at a constant rhythm, controlling the time with your watch. Only when you begin walking 50 blocks (3 miles/5 km) at this rhythm can you go on to the next level.

Energetic walking

In this case, the speed is intensified. The objective is to walk, three times per week, 10 blocks (1,100 yards/1,000 meters) in 9 to 10 minutes, with the goal of trying to walk 30 to 50 blocks. (To work up speed its best to swing your arms alternately). At this pace one burns a good amount of energy.

Aerobic walking

This consists of walking at high speed. The method consists of walking 10 blocks (1,100 yards/ 1,000 meters) in 6 to 8 minutes. The results of this exercise are excellent for losing weight, increasing your cardiovascular strength and reducing stress. Aerobic walking burns as many calories (nearly 300) as running, at the same time helping you get into great shape.

Your steps should be fast and energetic, with your arms swinging and bent at a 90 degree angle to help you pick up your pace.

As with all aerobic exercises, you need a greater amount of oxygen, which increases your lungs' capacity. This benefits your blood vessels, preventing the accumulation of fats and improving your heart function (see *Aerobic activity* box, on page 33).

PRE-WORKOUT STRETCH

Before and after you exercise, even with easy, light physical activity, including a simple walk, you should always take a few minutes to do stretching exercises to flex and relax your back.

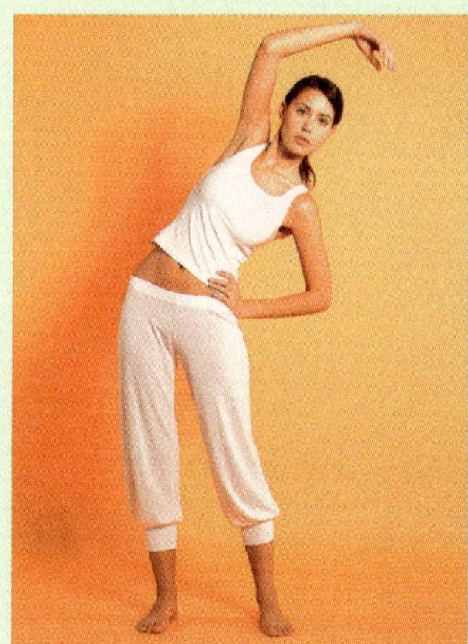

BACK STRETCH

With your feet shoulder width apart, lift up an arm and place your other hand on your hip. Lean to the side where your arm is placed on the hip, to form an arch. Stay in this position for 10 seconds, breathing deeply. Repeat with the other arm.

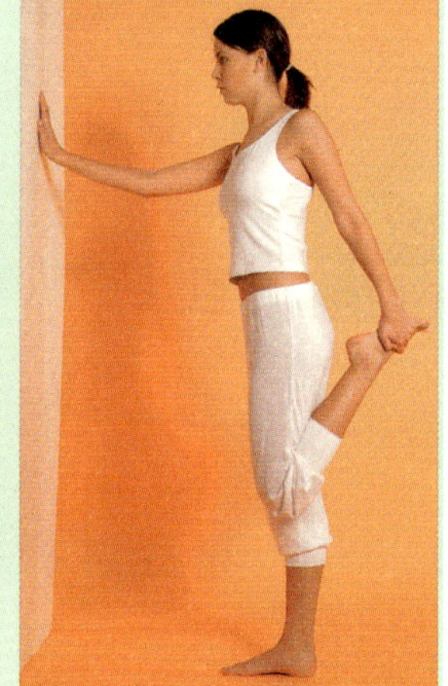

STRETCHING YOUR LEGS

Place your right arm stretched out on a wall or tree. With your left hand wrap your hand around your left foot and bring it to your buttocks. You should feel your quadriceps muscles stretching. Stay in this position for 10 to 20 seconds. Repeat with your other leg.

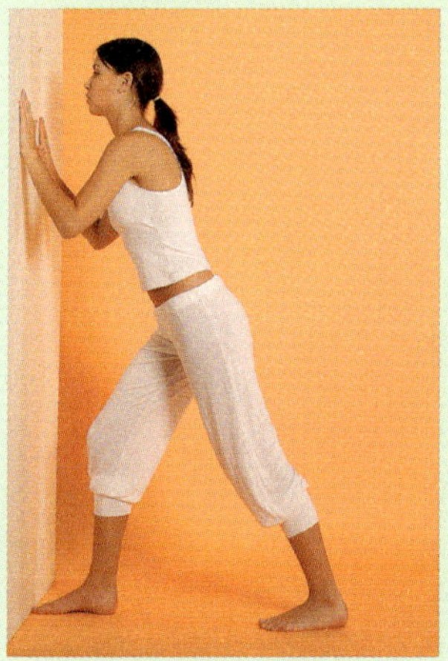

STRETCHING YOUR ANKLES AND HEELS

Against a wall or tree, bring your right foot some 12 in/30 cm in front of the other. Lean forward, bending your knee forward and keeping your hands against the wall. Your leg should stay stretched out, so that you feel that your joints are elongated. Your feet should remain firmly on the ground during this exercise. Stay in this position for 15 to 30 seconds, release and repeat with your other leg.

Gym activities

No matter your age or weight, you can always exercise to improve your health. You only need to keep in mind that for overweight people, working out too intensely or with high impact sports, can cause damage to your joints, knees, ankles and waist.

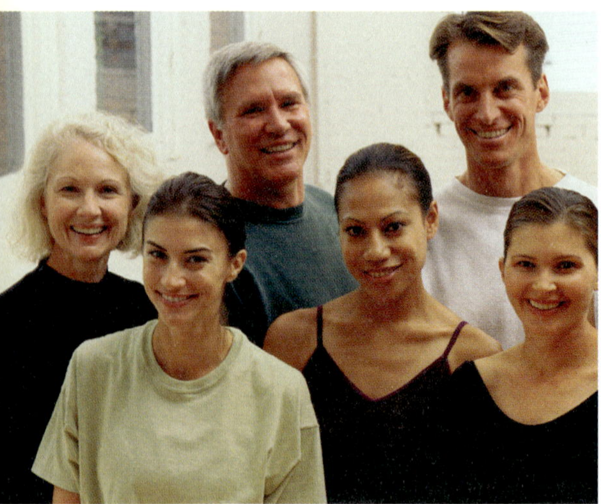

✚ At the gym there are a number of controlled activities that imitate, with computerized equipment, some exercises that we normally do outside, like walking or biking. Treadmills or stationary bikes are a recommended option for people who want to lose weight with minimal risk of injuries.

■ **Treadmill.** This computerized gym equipment improves your posture while walking and regulates your rhythm. You can easily track and control the progress you've made. It's important to follow a regular routine, preferably with a physical trainer. Exercising on gym equipment works the cardiorespiratory system. While you increase your stride you are also increasing the amount of oxygen your body needs. As a result your heart and lungs get aerobic exercise, while you are burning calories and toning muscles. The basic technique for using a treadmill:

• Get on the treadmill and place your feet on the platform.

Start with a walking speed of 3 miles/5 km per hour (1,400 yards/1,250 meters every 15 minutes). Continue walking at this speed until you establish a coordinated and relaxed rhythm.

• After a few minutes, gradually increase the speed, keeping your posture and walking in a synchronized rhythm.

• Lower the speed as you are about to end. Use caution when getting off the treadmill. Don't forget to stretch out before and after walking.

• Consult a physical trainer about increasing the rhythm as you make progress.

■ **Stationary bike.** Biking is a great aerobic exercise for burning calories and keeping your body fit. But traffic, lack of time and the weather can make biking outdoors difficult. However, a stationary bike is a good substitute. From an aerobic point of view, biking on a stationary bike for 30 minutes is equivalent to biking for an hour outdoors. You burn the same amount of calories as with running or jogging.

While on a stationary bike, it's recommended to keep your back straight and your arms firm but relaxed so that your body can follow the peddling motion. It's best to ask a personal trainer what speed and resistance are convenient for you.

AM I STRAINING MY BODY TOO MUCH?

30 minutes of exercise daily is a basic level to keep you energized and to build up resistance to physical exercise. However, the intensity does have its setbacks. As you build up your stamina you may have the urge to push yourself. You should keep in mind that exercising should not cause injuries, fatigue or pain. You should feel energized and healthy after a workout.

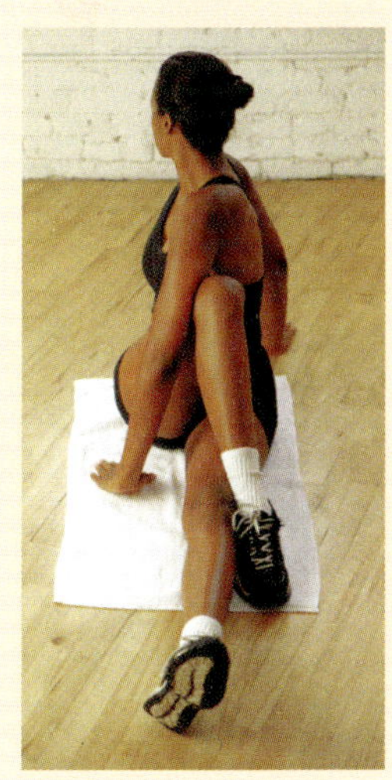

Water exercises

Swimming and exercising in the water (from water aerobics to running in water) are great for your body, bringing a number of health benefits at the same time helping you lose weight with little effort.

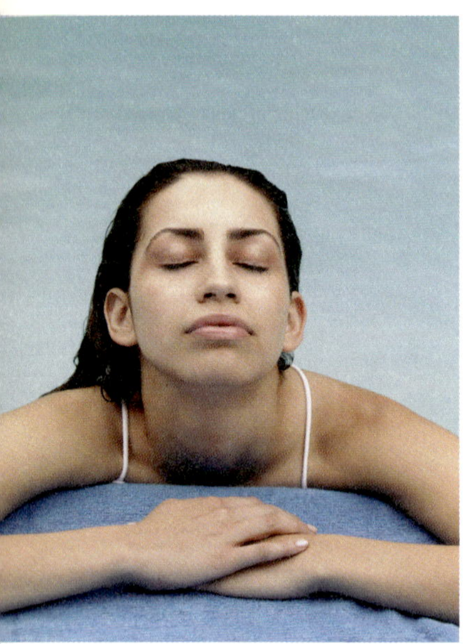

Exercising in water is an excellent way for people at whatever age or in any physical shape to workout with little risk of injuries. Water aerobics, which is done in a pool, indoor or outdoor, is a very valuable exercise for people who need a physical activity that's non-aggressive but challenging at the same time. Water aerobics increases your body's strength and flexibility while at the same time increasing your aerobic capacity, toning your muscles and improving your posture and coordination.

- **Swimming.** This is one of the most complete sports, because it uses almost every muscle in your body. It's also a "low impact" physical activity, but water provides 12 times more resistance than air, helping to relieve the impact of your body's weight. Moving in water tones your muscles while at the same time improving your muscle mass, with less risk of suffering from injuries from sudden movement. While at the same time, swimming is a psychologically gratifying exercise, because it's practiced in a pleasant environment, while the water's temperature can help you relax.

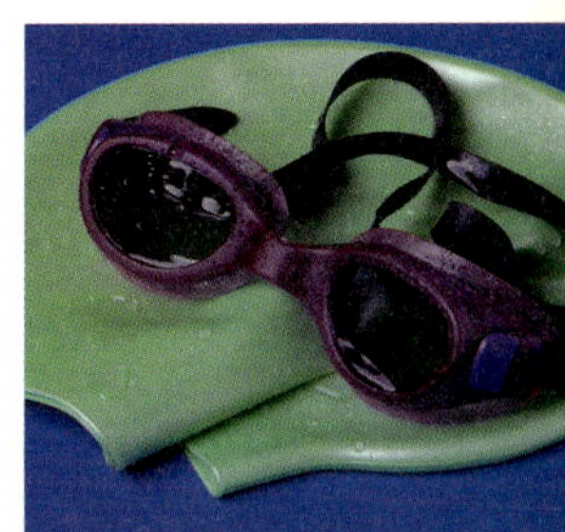

For swimming to be effective it's important to:

- Continue with your exercise routine to benefit from long-term results.
- Don't try to push yourself too far, swim according to your physical level.
- Keep a steady rhythm according to your physical state and remember to have fun.

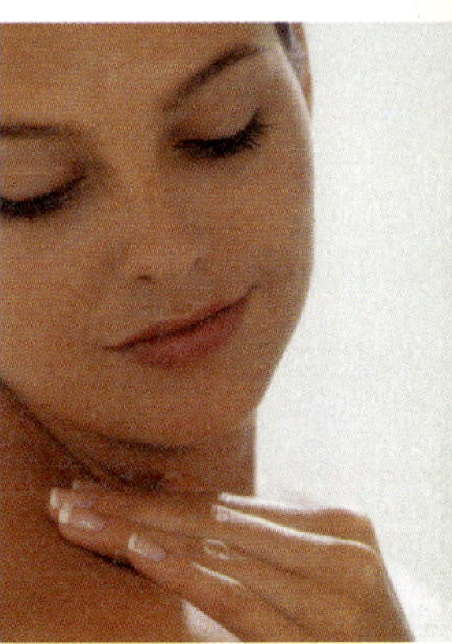

To have fun with swimming it's advised to:

- Follow health recommendations to prevent catching any infections.
- Control the water's temperature so that it's comfortable according to the weather and metabolism of each person.
- Make sure to keep your body hydrated and skin moisturized, to avoid skin problems.
- Protect your eyes to prevent irritation.

Water aerobics. This exercise provides similar benefits to swimming, it works certain muscles using the water for resistance. It's an ideal exercise for those who suffer from joint and back problems, while at the time it's a fun and relaxing sport.

AT THE LATTER STAGE OF LIFE

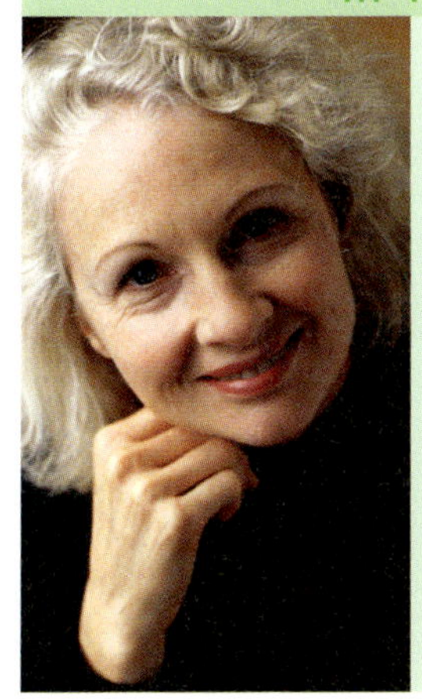

This is an age where it's important to keep up your physical activity, even if it's not an exercise plan. If you suffer from any of the following conditions (or all of them), it's important that you begin physical therapy to help you become more active:

- You can't get up from your chair without help.
- It's difficult for you to walk around the park with your grandchildren.
- You can't balance yourself on one leg.

It's important to consult your physician or to start physical therapy with gentle exercises that help strengthen your muscles, bones and joints, while making them more flexible. Do these exercises regularly, although at times it's difficult because you're tired or sore, because in the long run it will help to improve your health and the overall quality of your life.

Reducing pilates

This exercise uses a program of holistic stretching that helps to prevent and reduce weight gain through controlling your breathing and strength, and concentrating on your center of energy.

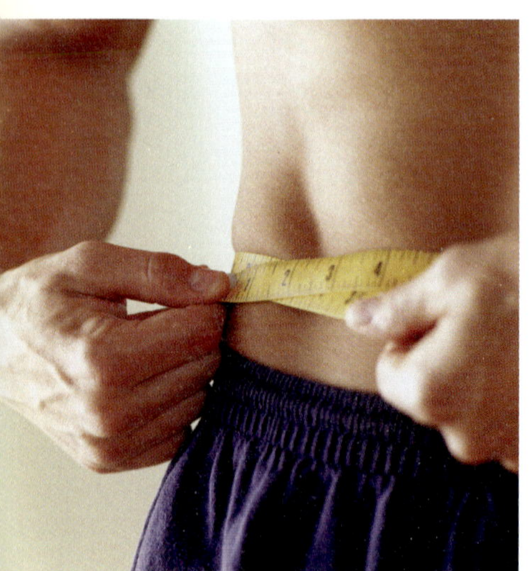

Pilates is a conditioning form of controlled movements that improves your strength and flexibility without building big muscles. Pilates can help you lose weight by toning your body and conditioning your muscles, especially in the center zone where some tend to build up fatty tissue. It uses the non-impact exercises devised by Joseph Pilates to develop strength, flexibility, balance and physical awareness.

THE FOUNDER

Founded by Joseph H. Pilates, around seventy years ago, it has recently gained new interest among chiropractics, physical therapists and anybody recovering from soft tissue injuries. Born in Germany in 1880, Joseph H. Pilates had a lifelong interest in body conditioning. As a frail child dedicated to becoming stronger, he later grew to become an accomplished skier, diver, gymnast, and boxer. At the outbreak of World War I, Pilates was interned as an "enemy alien" with other German nationals in England. During his internment, he refined his ideas and trained other internees in his system of exercise. He rigged springs to hospital beds, enabling bedridden patients to exercise against resistance, an innovation that led to his later equipment designs. An influenza epidemic struck England in 1918, killing thousands of people, but not a single one of Pilates' trainees died. This, he claimed, testified to the effectiveness of his system. He opened a fitness studio in New York and continued to train clients at his studio until his death in 1967 at the age of 87. Today, five million Americans practice Pilates, and the numbers continue to grow all over the world.

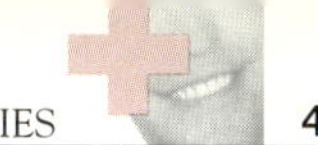

One hundred

Lying on your back, with your spine straight and your arms relaxed to the sides of your body. First bend your knees slightly and bring them up to hip level. Stretch out your legs and place the soles of your feet on the floor.

Inhale and as you exhale lift up your legs, together, a few inches from the ground. Bring your chin to your chest, without touching and keeping your head in this position. Lift up your arms a few centimeters. Next, move them, coordinating with your breathing. Inhale through the nose and exhale through the mouth five times. While moving your arms the same amount of times. Continue until you reach the number that's the name of the exercise: 100!

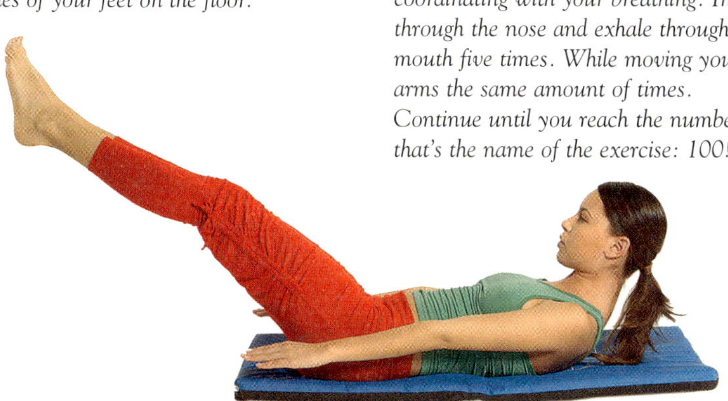

Roll forward

Lying down on your back with your arms stretched out behind your head and your legs straight and together. Inhale and as you exhale, lift your arms up. Inhale and, as you exhale lift up your neck and shoulders and bend over your belly button, continuing to move forward. Continue to move forward over your legs until your hands are at your feet, leave your arms parallel with your legs; see if you can wrap your hands around your toes. In this position, relax. Try to make the back longer with each outbreath. Next, come back to a sitting position, feeling how your spine is stretching. Exhale and lower your back (curved) until you are in the first position. Repeat four times.

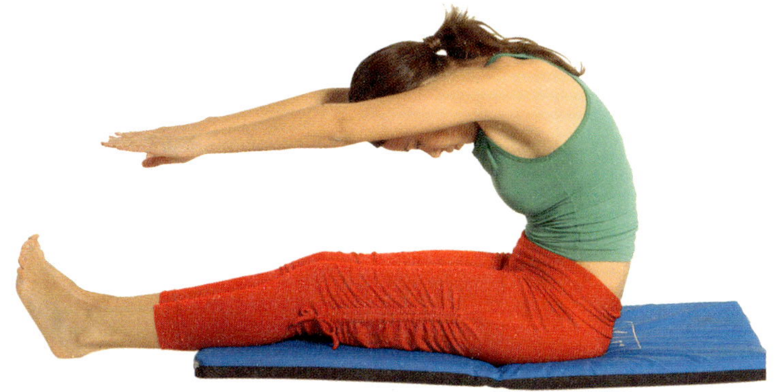

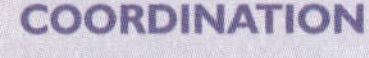

COORDINATION

To strengthen your muscles, you need to "surprise" them, with different movements. So they don't get accustomed and lose agility. Your breathing should coordinate with your movements.

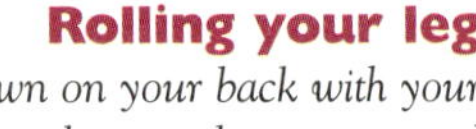

Rolling your leg

Lie down on your back with your spine on the mat, but not pressed against it. Inhale; as you exhale lift up your leg trying to align it with your knee and hip. Lastly, trace a semi-circle with this leg, from left to right above your body. Repeat six times with each leg.

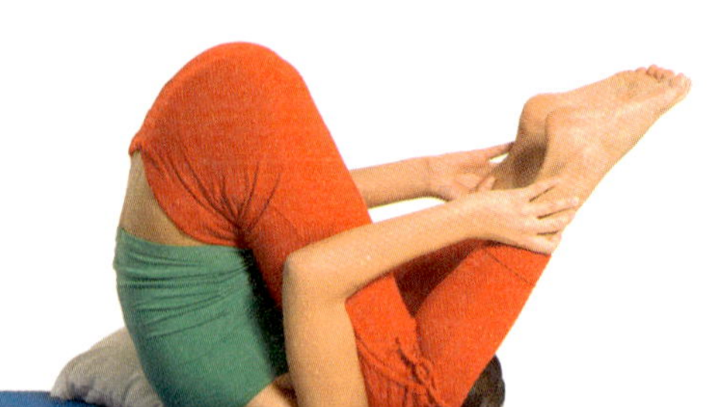

Rocking chair

In a seated position, seated straight on a mat. Keep the abdomen relaxed. Bend your knees and take hold of your ankles, bringing them close to your buttocks. Bring your forehead to your knees. Inhale; as you exhale, cave in your abdomen and rock backward. Leave your head between your knees, without forcing your body. You should concentrate on your abdomen when doing this movement. Continue rocking forward. Repeat six times.

Stretching your leg

Lying down on your back, with your ankles together and your toes pointed outward. Inhale; as you exhale lift up your neck and shoulders. Bend your right knee into your chest and wrap your arms around them. Lift up your left leg a few centimeters, keeping it completely straight. Repeat five times on each leg.

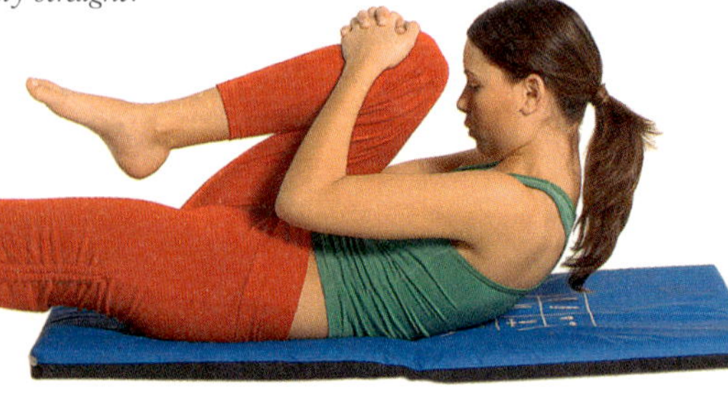

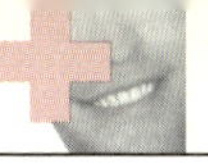

Stretching both legs

Lying down on your back with your spine relaxed, (not pressed against the mat, nor lifted up from it). Your arms and legs should be stretched out, ankles together and toes pointed forward. Inhale; as you exhale lift up (all at the same time) your neck, shoulders, arms and legs stretched out, trying to stretch them out even further. Inhale, as you exhale bend your knees, wrap your hands around your ankles and keep your legs to your chest, keeping your head in the same position. Repeat six times.

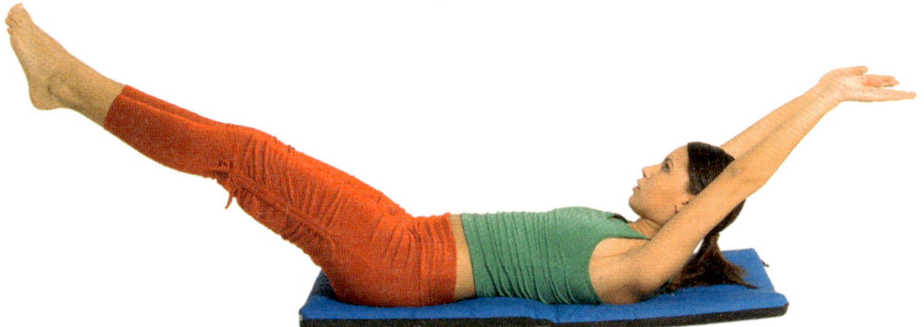

Forward backstretch

In a seated position with your back straight and your legs to the sides of your body. The palms of your hands should be on the mat. Your legs separated hip width and your toes pointed toward the ceiling. Lift your arms forward and place your hands on your knees. Inhale; as you exhale start to lower your back, keep it curved forward, bringing your forehead toward your knees. Curve your belly and continue to lower as much as you can, until your arms are parallel with your legs. Exhale and return to the initial position. Repeat six times.

THE BENEFITS OF PILATES

Pilates is an exercise routine that unifies the body and mind. The smooth, steady movements quiet your mind and soothe your nervous system. The body is strengthened and toned, posture is improved. Stress and exhaustion diminishes and sleep improves. With regular practice the mind gains a better clarity and sense of well-being. Each session involves movements that work the entire body, using deep muscles and oxygenating and detoxifying the body.

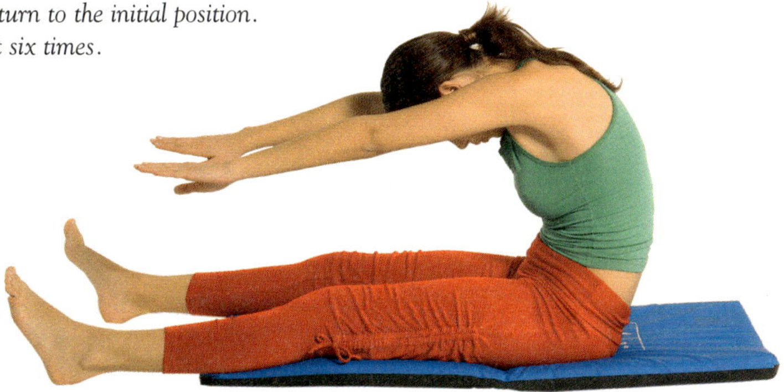

Shiatsu against hunger

According to the discipline of *shiatsu* there are a number of exact points on the body that, when pressure is applied to them, help to reduce anxiety and the sensation of hunger. These are simple techniques that you should use periodically.

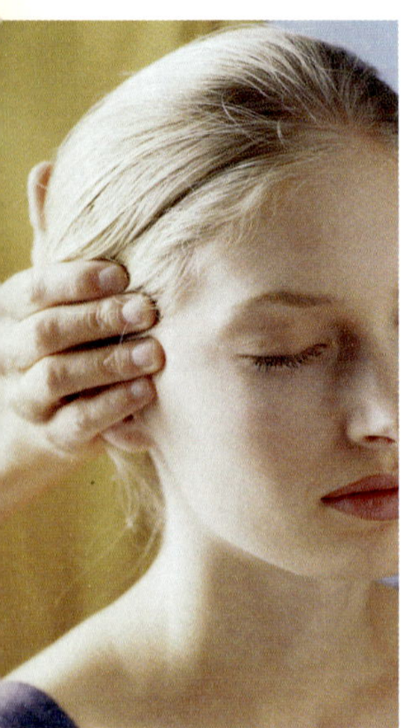

Shiatsu is a healing discipline based on ancient Oriental philosophy. Although this technique dates back more than 6,000 years, it's new for Western cultures. *Shiatsu* was recently introduced to the West in the 20th century. The method uses finger pressure on points or meridians that run along the body to balance the body's energy. This practice may be beneficial in cases of overweight, because applying pressure on specific points may help to reduce the appetite, while at the same time improving relaxation and relieving the anxieties that make you eat compulsively.

TO CONTROL YOUR HUNGER

Pressing on certain points helps to suppress hunger permitting prolonged periods between meals and the reducing of serving sizes.

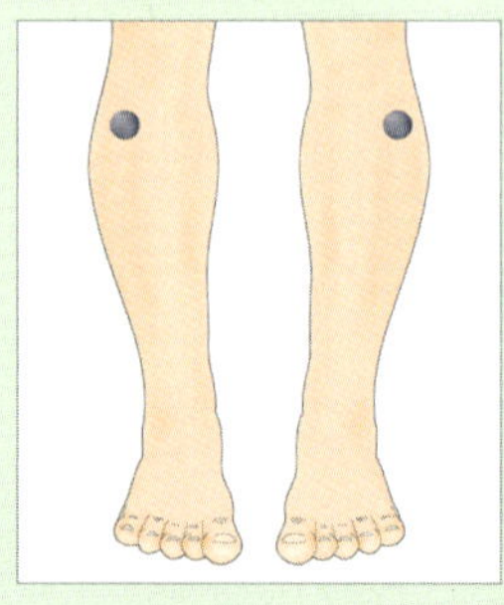

On the legs

If you apply pressure to the point that is the equivalent of a hand width apart from underneath the knee, in the hollow spot between the shin and calf, this may help to reduce the sensation of hunger, especially if it is applied in combination with the following pressure point.

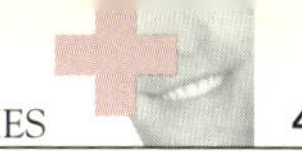

On the ankle

Press on the point that is the equivalent of a hand width distance from the internal edge of the bone on the inner ankle. This may help to reduce the sensation of hunger, especially if it is applied in combination with the previous pressure point.

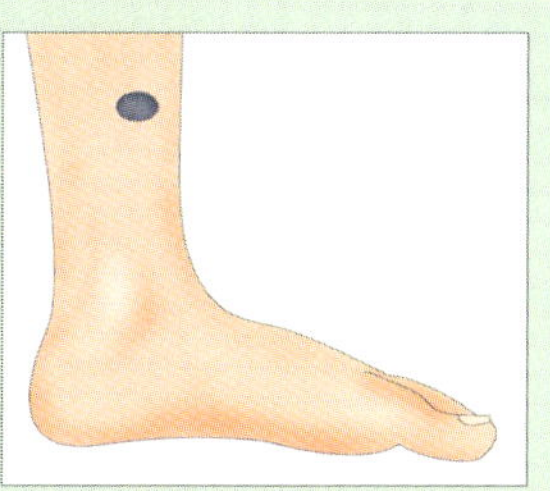

TO REDUCE ANXIETY

Applying pressure on the following points may help to relax and balance emotional levels for people who are overweight.

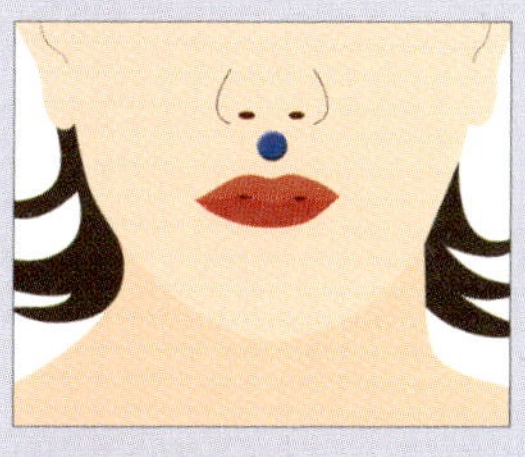

On the lip

To relax and calm hunger, press on the hollow between your upper lip and nose.

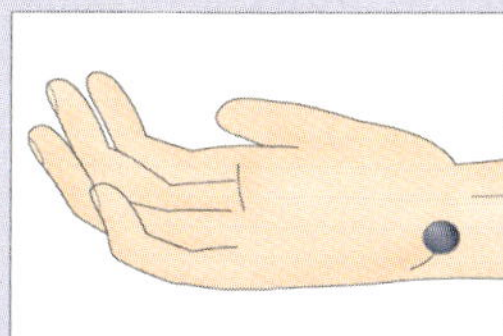

On the wrist

Activate the point located on the edge of the inner part of your wrist that's aligned to your pinkie finger.

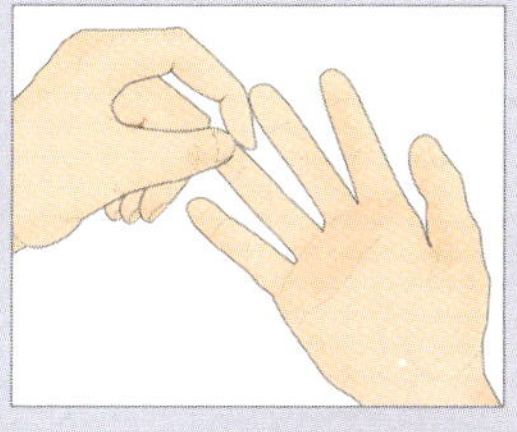

On the fingers

Massage your fingertips with your thumb. Next apply pressure on each fingertip, inhale and release the pressure as you exhale. After exhaling move on to the next fingertip.

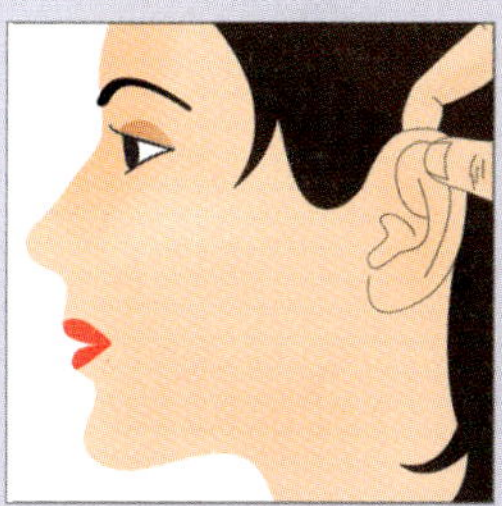

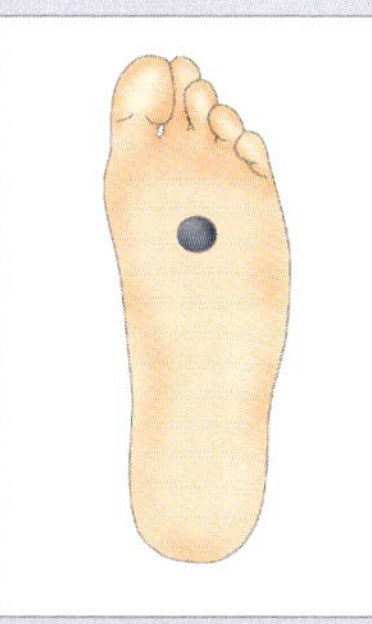

On the foot

Apply pressure on the point connected to the nervous system, located in the middle of the sole of the foot.

On the ears

Using your thumb and index finger, apply pressure along your outer ear. Apply pressure for a few seconds and then release.

Yoga for weight loss

Practicing yoga consistently and systematically improves relaxation and the union between the mind, body and spirit, to reduce the anxiety that makes us overeat. Among these benefits, physical yoga also contributes to a weight loss plan.

The postures or *asanas* for helping weight loss can be divided into three categories: those that massage the fatty tissue; those that affect the thyroid glands and those that help relaxation, diminishing the stress which can contribute to weight gain.

AGAINST FATTY TISSUE

The Crane and Half seated bend are poses that favor muscle tone and fight against fatty tissue.

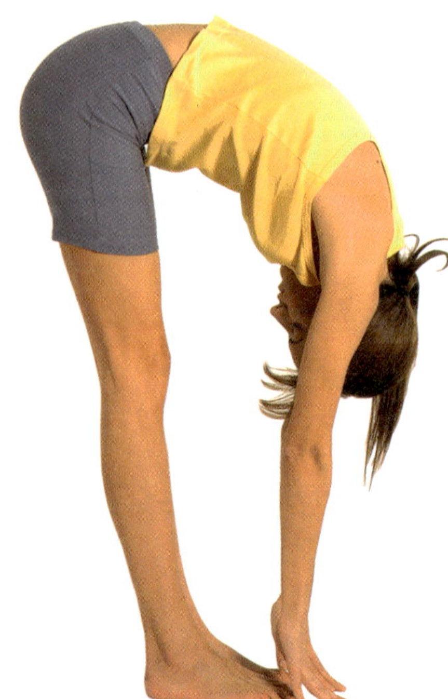

The Crane

This posture is similar to the Seated forward bend, but done standing. Bringing similar benefits. This exercise massages the abdominal muscles and fatty tissue. It helps to prevent fat from accumulating. It also stretches the spinal column and back muscles.

Standing on your feet, looking straight ahead with your arms to the sides of your body, take a deep breath. When you exhale, lower your torso straight down. Bring your arms to the floor, and if you can, place the palms of your hands on the ground. Try to bring your forehead to your knees. Keep breathing comfortably and with the abdomen tight, bring your torso down lower. Next, lift your torso up bit by bit. With your arms loose and relaxed, feel how your torso lifts up, vertebrae per vertebrae. To avoid becoming dizzy when releasing, inhale and lift your arms over your head. Then exhale and bring them down.

GENTLE EXERCISE
Yoga is a discipline designed to improve your flexibility and harmony. The exercises use gentle movements without straining your body. When practicing the *asanas* remember not to strain yourself. There is no need to push yourself too far. Remember to use gentle movements and don't push your body into a pose. Trough time and willpower, you will improve your body's health naturally and get in tune with your body.

Half seated bend

This is one of the most complete yoga poses, it has similar benefits to the Seated forward bend because it belongs to the same family of yoga poses. This position helps to fight weight gain, because it stretches and massages fatty tissue and helps your body to charge with energy and your mind to relax. This posture increases the flexibility of your back, leg muscles and knee joints and helps to fight against excess weight.

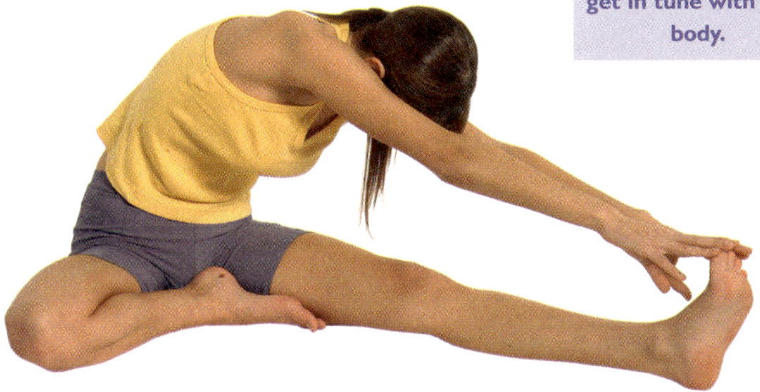

In a seated position, stretch out your left leg and bend your right leg, placing it on your inner left thigh so that your heel is touching your inner thigh. Keep your back straight and arms stretched. Take a deep breath and lift up your arms. While you exhale, lower your arms and torso over your left leg. Try to bring your forehead to your knee. Your hands should reach your ankle and if you can, the sole of your foot. Avoid unnecessary tension to lower all the way down. Continue breathing slowly. Stay in this position for as long as you feel comfortable. To release inhale and raise your arms. Then raise your torso. Exhale and lower your arms to your sides. Repeat with your other leg.

FOR THE THYROID GLANDS

There are two poses that benefit the thyroid glands: the Fish and the Cobra.

The Fish

This posture is highly beneficial for your body: it regulates thyroid and pineal gland functions. It also stretches your abdominal muscles, helping to treat overweight.

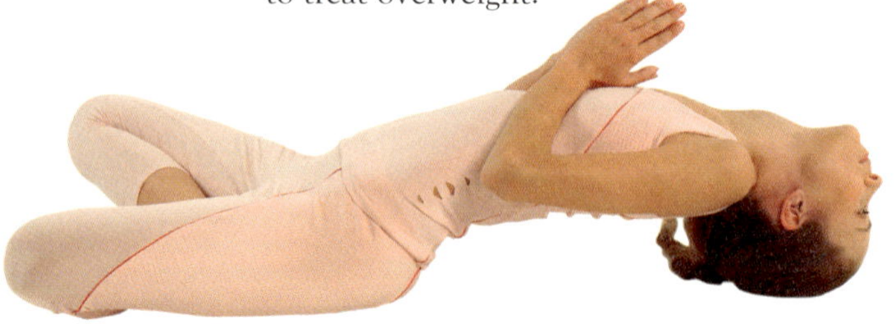

Sit on your heels, with your back straight, looking forward and your hands on your thighs. Breathing freely, bring your head all the way back, arching your back. Rest your weight on your elbows and palms of your hands. Drop your head back so that the top of your head is on the floor. You should feel how your vertebrae press together and the area around your throat opens. When you are firmly placed in this position, bring your hands to your chest and place the palms of your hands together. Stay in this position for as long as you find comfortable. To come out of the pose, place your elbows on the floor, inhale, bring your chin to your chest and roll on to your right side while you exhale.

The Cobra

This *asana* is beneficial for the body because it regulates the suprarenal glands' function, strengthens the back, increases the flexibility of the spine and helps to tone the abdominal muscles. In addition, it helps to increase your energy and to lift up your self-esteem. It helps to purify your body, important aspect when losing weight.

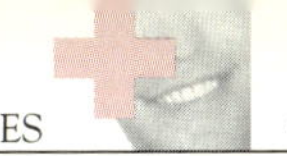

Lie down with your legs together and your forehead rested on the floor. Your legs should be straight with the front of your feet resting on the floor. Place your elbows, forearms and the palms of your hands on the floor. The palms of your hands should stay at the same height as your shoulders and your head should be slightly pressed against the floor. Contract your buttocks and lift up your chest, slowly so as not to harm the lower back. Extend your arms at the same time as you lift up your chest. If this causes any discomfort, don't strain yourself and keep your head looking forward. To release, slowly lower your body while you place on the ground: the abdomen, and lastly the chest, always stretched forward. Next, bring your chin to your chest and rest one cheek on the ground.

TO RELAX

To relax we recommend the *Sitali* breathing and Deep or diaphragmatic breathing.

Sitali breathing exercise

This exercise helps to calm hunger and thirst. It helps to purify your blood and improve sleep.

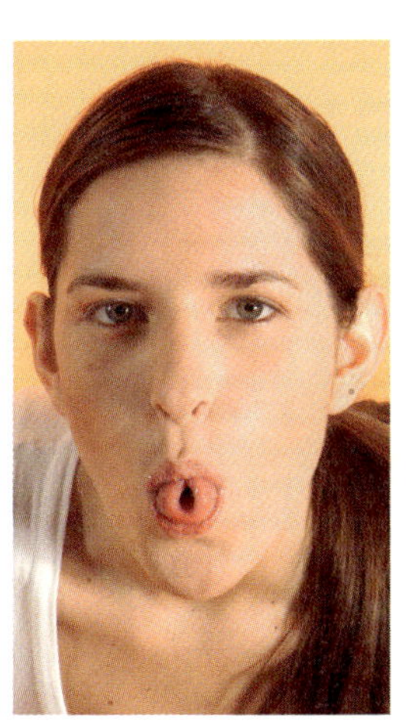

Stick out your tongue, so that the tip is over your lips. Fold your tongue to form a "tube" and breathe through your tongue. You will note that the air cools off your tongue. Continue inhaling in this pose for as long as you feel comfortable. Next, exhale through your nose.

DEEP OR DIAPHRAGMATIC BREATHING

Newborns use this breathing, which is the perfect breath. This breathing technique is a source of life that helps to calm your mind and control the anxiety that causes overeating. It lifts up your spirit, relieving the depression usually accompanied with overweight. It balances the nervous system, energizes and relaxes the muscles. It also helps to bring oxygen and purify the blood. It is called diaphragm breathing, because it uses this muscle.

- It's best to practice this technique lying down on the floor or on a padded mat. However, advanced practitioners can do this exercise sitting or standing up with their back straight.
- Take in deep breaths without your chest lifting up but from the abdomen. You should inhale slowly to fill the lungs; you should exhale completely before inhaling again.
- As the air passes through the throat you can press on the esophagus to produce a sound similar to snoring.
- Repeat 4 or 5 complete cycles.

Essential nutrients

Some say, "you are what you eat." In some ways this is true. Our physical and mental health depends on how many nutrients we are getting from our daily diets.

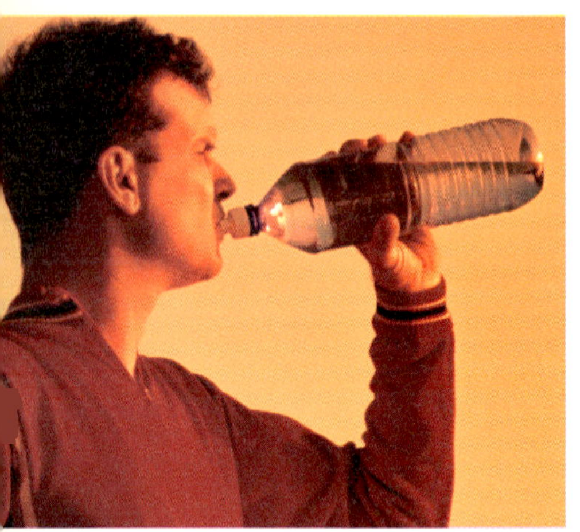

A basic and essential nutrient is water, the most important element for our bodies after oxygen. We need between 8 to 10 glasses of water daily, which we get from the foods and drinks we consume.

We need water to transport nutrients and waste through our bodies and to release toxins through sweat and urine. Water is a principal component of the fluids that our bodies use for digestion; it helps to regulate our body temperatures and to keep the digestive system functioning correctly.

HEALTHY CALORIES

Calories come from carbohydrates or glucides, proteins and fats or lipids. These nutrients must arrive to the body in the appropriate proportions.

• **50 to 55** % of calories should come from carbohydrates, with most of these coming from special carbs that are called "complex carbohydrates". These are absorbed slowly and generally contain fiber. Complex carbohydrates are found in **whole grain cereals** and derivatives (such as flour and baked goods without fats),

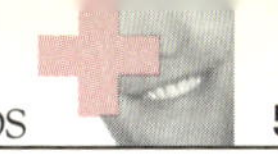

beans and derivatives, **starchy vegetables** (potato, sweet potatoes, cassava, corn), and other **fruits** and **vegetables**.

- **15 to 20 %** of calories should come from low-fat proteins. For example: **lean meats, egg whites, hard cheeses** and **skim dairy products** and also **beans**.
- **30 %** of calories should come from fats made up of healthy fatty acids. The healthiest type of fats are monounsaturated –**olive, corn, canola oils**– can be eaten. Our bodies also need saturated fats –animal derived fats– but should be eaten in moderate quantities because saturated fats over time can block heart arteries.
- Polyunsaturated fats –oils from seeds and nuts– are also healthy, but should be eaten in moderation, because they oxidize easily and wear out cellular membranes. For this group the following are especially recommended: **dried nuts, avocado, seeds**.

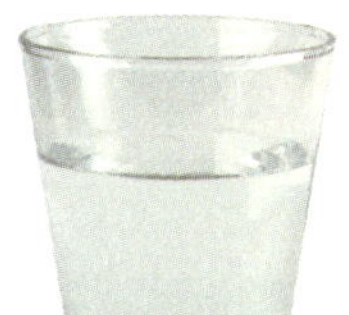

FOR WATER

When talking about drinking sufficient liquids, nutritionists advise to drink water. You can complement water consumption with fruit and vegetable juices and infusions. Freshly squeezed fruit and vegetable juices are healthy and rich in vitamins, minerals and antioxidants.

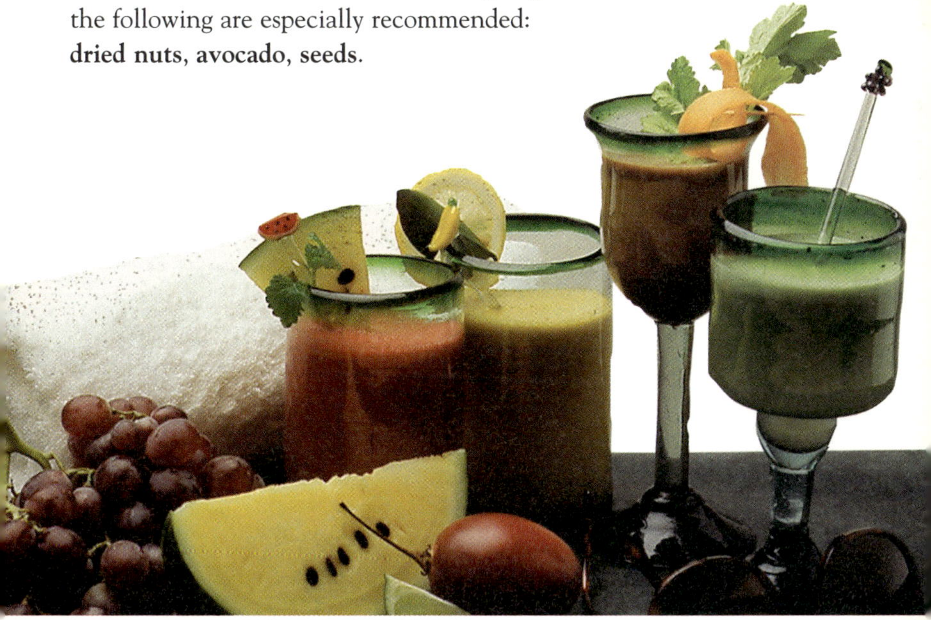

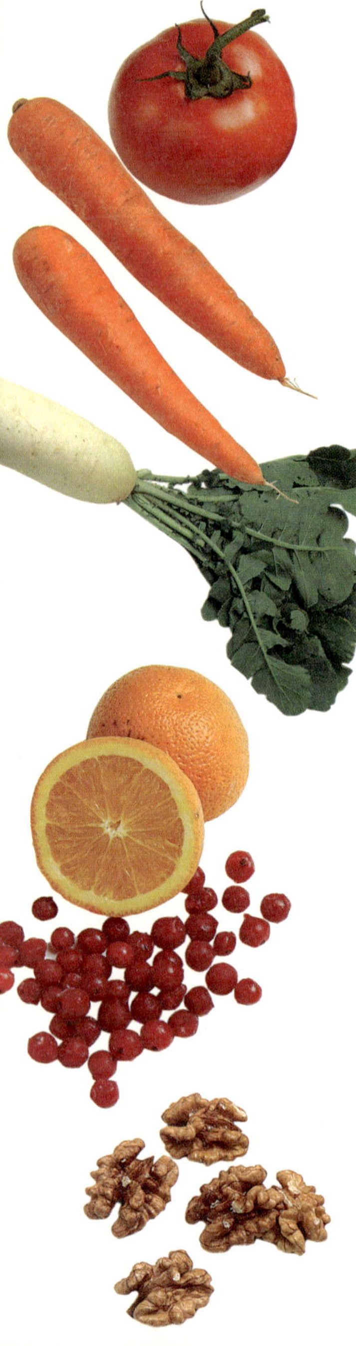

FIBER

Our body needs fiber daily, at least 1 oz/ 30 g per day. Insoluble fiber (in water) benefit intestinal health; soluble fibers help aid in metabolism; because they improve the absorption and breakdown of sugars and fats in the blood, helping to reduce blood cholesterol levels. To get the minimum recommended dose of fiber it's recommended eating **whole grains**, **beans** and plenty of **fruits** and **vegetables**.

MINERALS

These are essential for the formation of the organs and tissues that support the multiple functions vital for the body.

- **Calcium.** A basic nutrient for healthy bones and teeth, as well as supporting nerve transmission and muscular movement. It's necessary to get at least 1,000 mg of calcium per day; you can easily get high quality calcium through the consumption of **dairy products**, but also in **dried nuts**, **seeds**, **barley**, **fish with small bones** (**sardines**).
- **Iron.** Forms part of red blood cells and helps to transport oxygen to body tissues. Iron derived from meats are the best absorbed. Iron from **green leafy vegetables**, **beans**, **eggs** and **fortified foods** is absorbed less easily. It's recommended eating iron rich foods together with other foods that contain vitamin C.
- **Sodium.** This mineral is absorbed in the body through **table salt** and a number of prepared foods (**bread**, **crackers**, **breakfast cereals**, **cheeses** and **deli meat**).

It's important to avoid eating excess sodium, because it can increase your risk for high blood pressure and edema. Prioritizing fresh foods and seasoning with plenty of herbs and spices decreases the amount of salt used in cooking, while keeping foods flavorful.

■ **Potassium.** It's important to get enough potassium, because it protects the body against high blood pressure. It's best to eat plenty of **fresh fruits** and **vegetables**.

■ **Magnesium.** This mineral regulates with calcium to keep the bones and teeth healthy. It also keeps the neuromuscular system balanced. It is found in **whole grains**, **deep green leafy vegetables**, **fish** and **meat**, **seeds** and **dried nuts**.

■ **Zinc.** This mineral also contributes to the health of the bones, skin and hair, as well as increasing the defenses against free radicals. It is present in **dairy products**, **meats** and **grains**.

■ **Selenium.** This is an important antioxidant for protecting body tissue. It also fortifies the action of the antioxidant vitamin E. It is found in **beans**, **fish**, **dried fruits**, **nuts** and **cabbage family vegetables**.

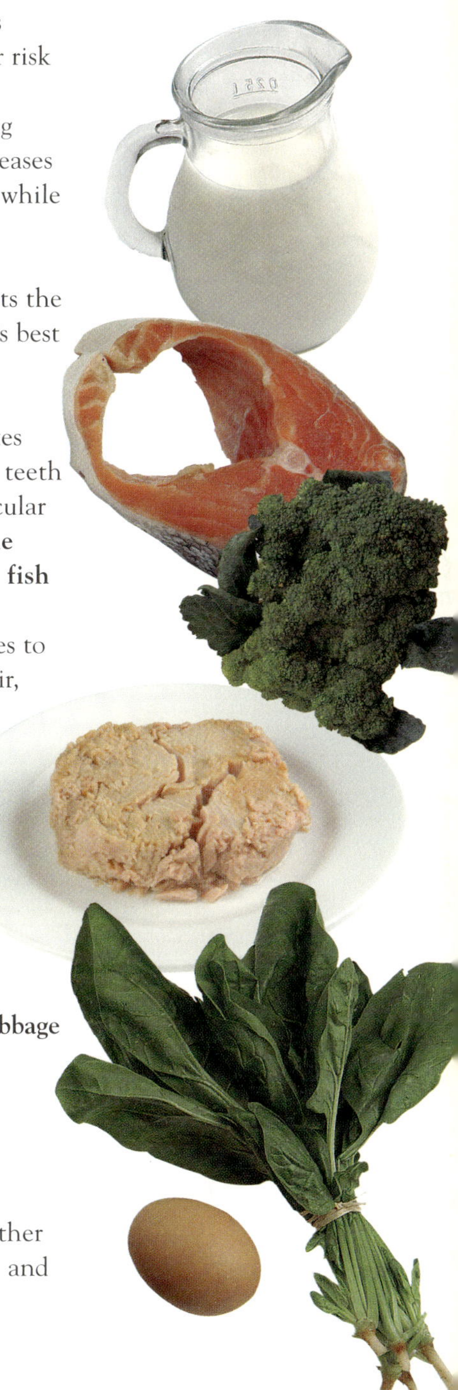

VITAMINS

All vitamins are vital for the body's health. For optimal absorption you should try to eat fresh vegetables, either raw or cooked. There are fat-soluble and water soluble vitamins.

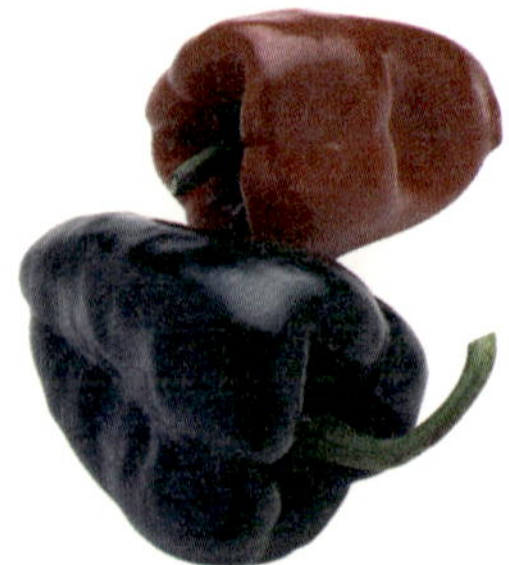

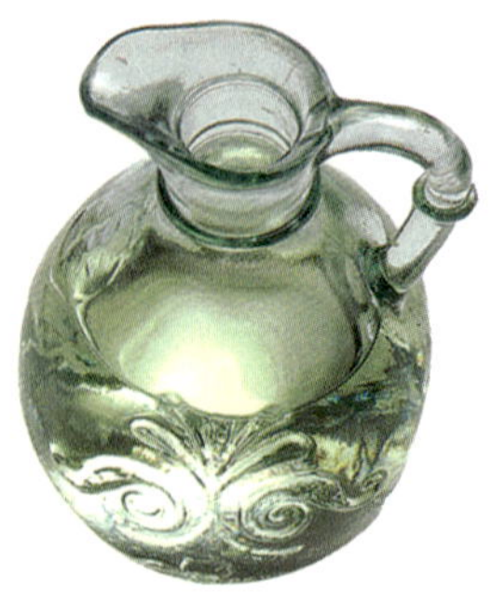

Fat-soluble vitamins need fatty acids for absorption, they also accumulate in fatty deposits in the body. The following are fat-soluble vitamins:

- **Vitamin A.** This vitamin helps to keep the skin and sight healthy. It protects the body against infections. Natural sources include: **dairy products**, **eggs**, **green veggies** and **red** and **orange vegetables**.
- **Vitamin E.** Strong antioxidant that helps in the formation of red blood cells. Found in **sunflower** and **corn oils**, **seeds** and **dried fruits**.
- **Vitamin D.** Supports the breakdown and absorption of calcium. Sunlight activates the synthesis of this vitamin in our bodies. It is found in **milk**, **yogurt**, **eggs** and **entrails**.

Water-soluble vitamins need water to be absorbed; they are flushed out of the system through urine, making daily intake of water-soluble vitamins a necessity. These vitamins aren't stored in the body.

- **Vitamin C.** Helps to keep body tissue strong and keep the hair healthy. It helps in the absorption of iron and acts as an active antioxidant. It is found in **citrus fruits**, **kiwi**, **tomatoes**, **peppers** and **cabbage family vegetables**.
- **Vitamin B_1.** Helps to keep the nervous system and brain active and healthy. This vitamin is fundamental for proper metabolism of carbohydrates. It is found in **whole grain cereals** and

derivatives, **wheat germ**, **brewer's yeast** and **meat** (especially in **pork**).

- **Vitamin B_2.** Essential for the skin's health and eyesight. It supports metabolism. Natural sources are **dairy products**, **meat**, **dried fruits**, **nuts** and **beans**.
- **Vitamin B_3.** Protects the skin's health and the digestive system. It supports metabolism. All foods high in protein are natural sources: **meats**, **beans**, **cereals**, **dairy products** and **eggs**.
- **Vitamin B_{12}.** Fundamental for the development of red blood cells. Vegetarians should make sure to find alternative sources for this vitamin, because it is only found in animal derived products –**meats**, **eggs**, **dairy products** and specially **fortified cereals**.
- **Folic acid.** This vitamin is very important for the synthesis of DNA (making it an essential vitamin before conception and during the first months of pregnancy). Natural sources are **fresh green vegetables** or slightly cooked vegetables, **whole grains**, **beans** and **fruits**.
- **Beta carotenes.** These aren't exactly vitamins, but some are considered to be provitamin A and are all important natural antioxidants. They are found in **yellow** and **orange vegetables** such as **carrots** and **squash**. They are also found in some **red vegetables** such as **peppers** and **tomatoes**.

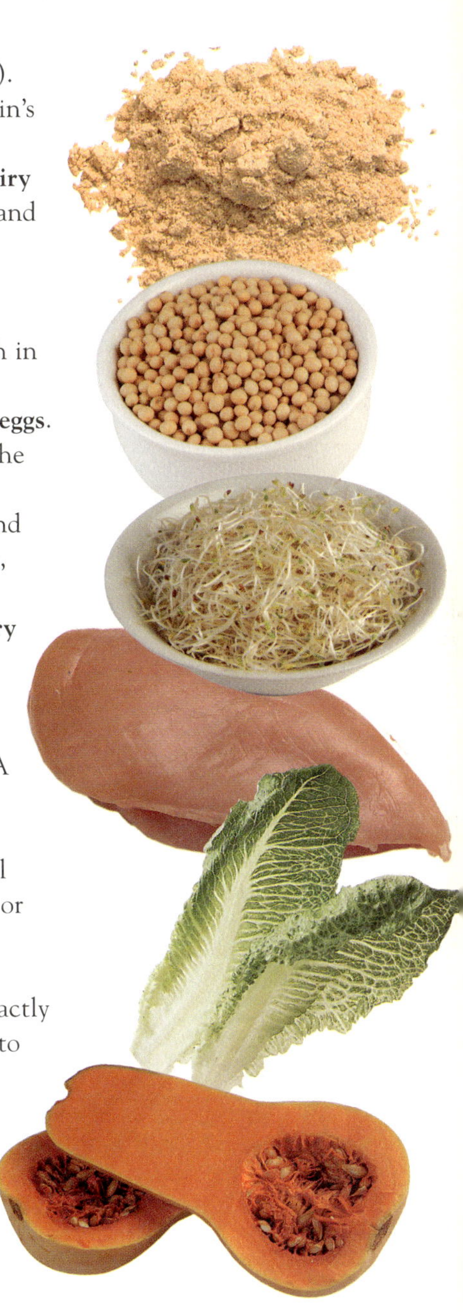

Natural help

Many herbs, in the form of teas and other preparations, can help to control hunger and anxiety. Some essential oils for topical use have similar benefits, also of natural origin, ideal for lifting the spirits and calming anxiety.

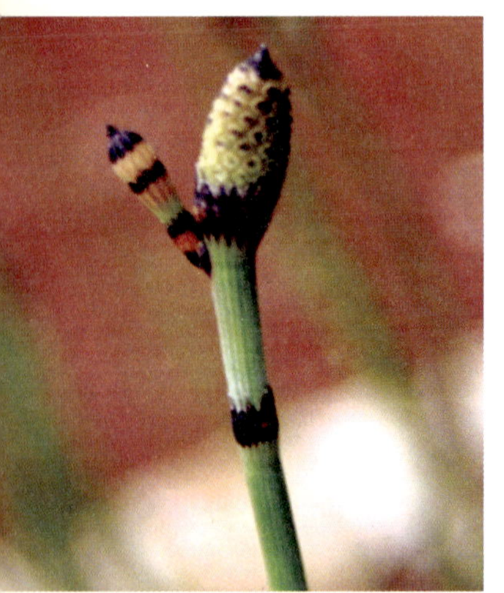

Nature offers infinite resources for controlling our weight and reducing fats, through relieving the anxiety that makes some people console their worries with food. Some medicinal plants can be found more easily than others depending on where you live.

Horsetail
(Equisetum sp)

- **Parts used.** The dried stems which have an aroma similar to camomile. It is used to prepare infusions and decoctions as well as to make tinctures.
- This herb has powerful diuretic properties. It helps to clean your urine tract (detoxifying action), it purifies the blood and may aid in weight loss.
- **Warning.** In cases of blood in the urine or

NOTE
You should always consult your physician before starting any herbal treatment.

DIURETIC DOSES

In infusion. *Place 2 teaspoons of horsetail in 1 cup with boiling water. Let steep for 15 minutes, drain and drink 2 or 3 times a day.*
In decoction. *Boil 2 teaspoons of horsetail in 1 cup of water over a low heat for at least 1/2 hour to extract its minerals. Drink 2 times a day. You can prepare a larger amount, and keep it in a jar in the refrigerator to drink cold.*
In tincture. *Take 2 teaspoons of horsetail tincture diluted in a glass of water 3 times a day.*

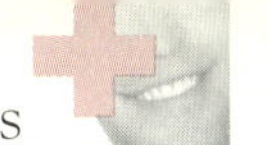

sudden changes in menstrual flow, consult your doctor. You should not use this herb during pregnancy.

Bladder wrack

(Fucus vesiculosus)

• **Parts used.** The entire plant, which is a dark brown algae. It can be used to prepare infusions; it can also be used in powder form, capsules and tinctures.

• It is a source of iodine and potassium. In the case of dysfunctional thyroid glands, iodine stimulates their secretion.

• Stimulates the metabolism and aids in weight loss, especially for cases of obesity with symptoms of fatigue.

• **Warning.** Do not administer to children under 5 years of age. You shouldn't take this herbal remedy during pregnancy or if you are breastfeeding. If you have thyroid gland dysfunction, you should use this herbal remedy under strict medical prescription.

RECOMMENDED DOSE

• **In capsules or tablets.** Take 1 bladder wrack tablet 3 times a day, or follow the instructions on the container, or consult your physician.

• **Dried.** Take 1 to 2 tablespoons daily, you can add it to your meal or soup.

• **In infusion.** Use 2 teaspoons in an infusion. Let steep for 3 to 4 minutes, until the infusion has taken on a deep color. Drink 1 to 2 cups daily. For children we recommend using half the dose.

ESSENTIAL OILS FROM A TO Z

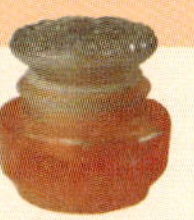

CLARY SAGE

In inhalations or massages, promotes well-being and balance. It can be used to help control your weight, because it tends to decrease hunger. It helps to bring on relaxing sleep, preventing late night snacking. You can add a few drops to a warm bath before going to bed, along with a few drops of geranium or lavender.

Safety. It can have sedative effects, making it difficult to concentrate. Do not operate heavy equipment or drive after using clary sage.

CYPRESS

This essential oil is used for inhalations or to aromatize the room when you are feeling the anxiousness that makes you feel hungry.

Safety. When using during massages, do not apply pressure to varicose veins. This oil could warm up the zone and cause discomfort.

WARNING

Essential oils are for external use **only**, they should **never** be ingested. Keep stored away from children and keep away from your eyes.

Gambooge

(Garcinina cambogia)

• **Parts used.** The flesh of the fruit and the bark, wich are used to make dry or liquid extracts.

• Hidroxycitric acid is obtained from the extracts of this plant, which is native to India. In the south of that country the bark is used in powder form as a condiment.

• It is a powerful agent against obesity, because the hidroxycitric acid blocks the synthesis of fatty acids and accelerate the burning of fats by the liver.

• Controls appetite, thus reducing food intake.

• Helps in treatement of overweight without affecting the muscle mass.

• There are not contra indications for its use.

GAMBOOGE FOR WEIGHT LOSS

Drink 25-30 drops of fluid extract 3 times per day. Where dry extract (powder) is used, take 2,000 mg (in pill or capsule form). Whether in fluid or dry form, gambooge must be taken before meals and must be consumed as part of a diet recommended by a doctor or dietary specialist.

Glucomannan

(Amorphophalus konjac)

• **Parts used.** The stems that grow under the ground are used to make capsules and powder.

• This plant comes from Southern China, Vietnam and Japan.

• This vegetable fiber is widely used in weight loss plans. It has the capacity to absorb 100 times its weight in water, producing a feeling of fullness.

• Like many soluble fibers, glucomannan can bind with a variety of substances in the digestive tract to slow digestion, relieve constipation and reduce the absorption of fat and carbohydrates.

• This herb increases the amount of

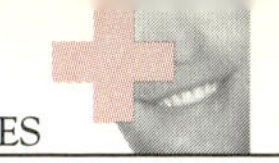

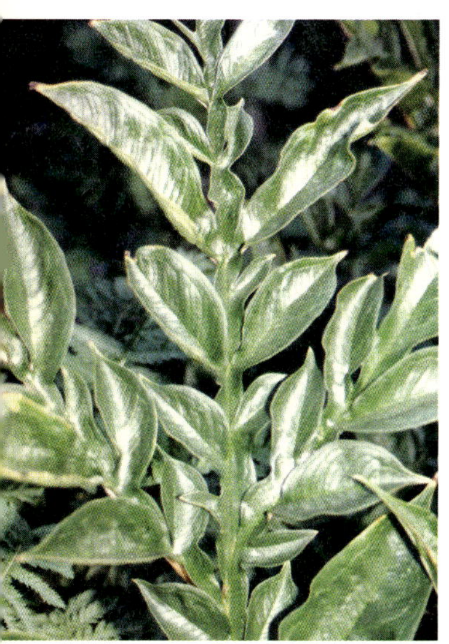

calcium and phosphorus in the bones. It is recommended for women in menopause, a stage in life where women generally gain weight and lose calcium mass in their bones. This herb also provides vitamin B_6, which helps to relieve premenstrual syndrome.

• Decreases the levels of cholesterol in the body, because it traps cholesterol in bile acids and increases excretion.

• **Warning.** This herb is not recommended if you suffer from stretched out or the narrowing of respiratory tract or digestive tract.

SLIMMING DOSE

• **In capsule or pill forms.** Take 1 or 2 capsules of glucomannan 500-750 mg with at least 2 glasses of water or juice 1/2 hour before meals.

• **Dried powder.** Dilute 1,500 mg of glucomannan powder in fruit juice. Slowly sip 1/2 hour before meals. Then drink 1 or 2 glasses of water.

Bitter orange

(Citrus aurantium)

• **Parts used.** The fruit, green or ripe and the flowers and leaves are used in infusions and decoctions. They are also used to make extracts and essential oils.

ESSENTIAL OILS FROM A TO Z

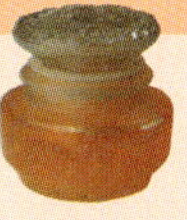

GERANIUM

This essential oil with its euphoric aroma is used in cellulitis fighting massages, because its properties help to increase circulation. A few drops in a hot bath can help you relax. A few drops in a tepid bath will revitalize you. Blended with bergamot it can help relieve the states of depression and nervousness that are common for overweight people.

Safety. You should always dilute geranium, because it can irritate the skin when used in pure form.

JUNIPER

Inhaling this aroma helps to clear the mind, lift up your spirits and increase your self-esteem, especially if you are overweight. When used in massages, it can help reduce cellulitis, because it relieves water retention in the body. To increase its properties you can blend it with geranium and grapefruit.

Safety. You shouldn't use juniper during pregnancy because this essential oil can induce labor.

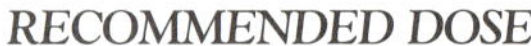

RECOMMENDED DOSE

- ***Infusion with leaves.*** *Let 1 teaspoon to 1 tablespoon of bitter orange leaves steep per 4 cups of boiling water. Drain and drink 2 to 3 cups per day.*
- ***Infusion with flowers.*** *Add 1/2 teaspoon of bitter orange flowers to 1 cup of boiling water. Let sit for 10 minutes. Drink 2 to 3 cups per day.*

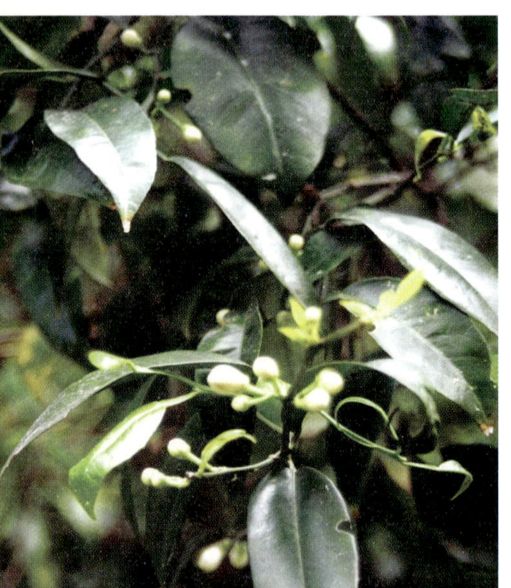

- Native to China, this plant's medicinal properties have been utilized since the Middle Ages by Arabic healers.
- This herb helps in weight loss, because it is a diuretic and stimulates digestion. It is also used as a sedative, calming the nervousness that may cause you to eat.
- This herb doesn't only induce weight loss, but also improves physical well-being. It also helps to tone the muscles.
- The green fruits have greater therapeutic properties than the ripe fruits.
- This plant contains vitamins A, B, C and flavonoids. It also contains synephrine, a component that has been proven to diminish the appetite without causing headaches. Many over the counter diet drugs contain isolated synephrine extracted from this plant.
- **Warning.** In some cases this herb can cause contractions during pregnancy. It shouldn't be used topically on children under 6 years

of age or for people who suffer from respiratory problems.

Green tea

(Camelia sinensis)

- **Parts used.** The stems and leaves are used in infusions.
- Green tea is made from the shoots of the *Camelia sinensis* tree, the same as common tea. The differences is in the amount of fermentation of these shoots.
- According to history, this spice was discovered by the Chinese Emperor Shen Nung. While taking a break in a hunting expedition, some green tea leaves fell into a pot where he was boiling water. The emperor was surprised by the drink's color and aroma. When he tried it he found that it was relaxing and invigorating.
- This tea is rich in minerals, vitamins A, B and C and volatile oils.

DIGESTIVE GREEN TEA

We recommend buying green tea in small quantities to guarantee freshness. To prepare boil 4 cups of water and let it cool for 5 minutes. Add the tea –1 teaspoon per cup– into the teapot, previously warmed with hot water. Pour the boiled water on top and let steep for 2 to 3 minutes. The sooner you drink the tea, the more stimulating the effect. However, if you wait more than 5 minutes, the tea will be more relaxing. Healthy dose: up to 3 cups per day.

ESSENTIAL OILS FROM A TO Z

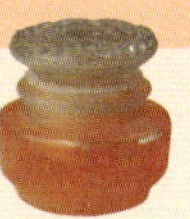

LAVENDER

This essential oil is recommended for weight control, because it helps relieve the symptoms of stress that may create the urge to overeat. Blended with marjoram it can have a calming effect.

Safety. This essential oil can cause drowsiness for people who suffer from low blood pressure. Do not use during pregnancy.

LEMON

Applying lemon essential oil externally helps to clear your mind, get over the hunger and emotional confusion related to weight gain. In massages it can help to fight cellulitis and to relieve varicose veins because it has decongestive properties.

Safety. Make sure to dilute this essential oil when using topically. It's best to avoid direct sunlight after using lemon essential oil because it increases your skin's photosensitivity.

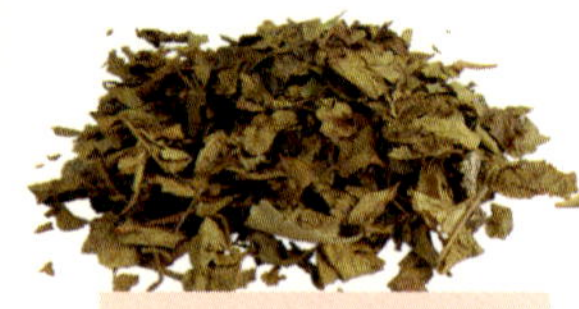

TIP

• Don't use special spoons for infusing tea, because the leaves become packed so that the components aren't released. The ideal is for the leaves to float in the water.

• Don't prepare a greater quantity than you will drink in an hour's time. However, depending on the variety of green tea used, you can reuse the leaves. A tablespoon can be used for 4 cups. If there's tea left after infusing, remove the leaves from the water, so they don't leave a bitter taste.

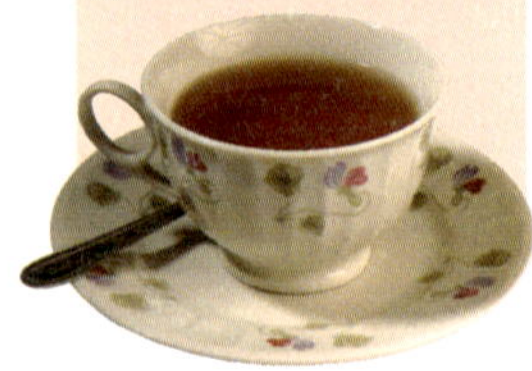

• Green tea is a powerful antioxidant. In addition, the tannins found in green tea have an astringent effect on the intestinal tract, helping to absorb nutrients and flush out impurities, helping in weight loss.

• **Warning.** Excessive amounts of tea can harm the liver, cause constipation, and because of its caffeine content, cause irritability and heart palpitations.

Yerba maté

(Ilex paraguariensis)

• **Parts used.** The leaves are used to make infusions or to make capsules and tinctures.

• This plant grows in South America, in the bordering region between Argentina, Brazil and Paraguay. The native indigenous people from this zone, the Guaraní, macerated the leaves for days and then drank the infusion as a remedy for a number of illnesses. They also used it as an elixir to energize and comfort.

• *Yerba maté* helps in weight loss, because of its chemical substances such as the xanthines and thermogenie found in it. They have lipolytic properties that allow the body to break down fat and turn it into energy.

• It is a natural diuretic and laxative. It is also a powerful stimulant. *Yerba maté* contains vitamins, including vitamin C, complex B vitamins, minerals such as potassium, calcium, magnesium and antioxidants.

THERAPEUTIC DOSE

• **In pill or capsule forms**. Generally, 2,000 mg taken in 2 to 3 doses to take advantage of its thermogenie effects to help you absorb fat.

• **In a tincture.** Use *yerba maté* drops as a tonic and diuretic. It's recommended 40 drops 3 times a day.

CORRECT WAY TO PREPARE MATÉ

This drink is very popular in many parts of South America. It is traditionally drank in a wood or metal container or gourd. A *bombilla* (metal filter straw) is used to sip the hot beverage.

To prepare the *yerba maté* infusion, place the dried minced leaves of *yerba maté* inside the *maté* cup, and moisten with cool water -let sit for a minute or so. Next add hot water, below boiling degree (approx. 158 °F/70 °C), this is called "cebar el mate". You can also substitute hot water for very cold water and lemon, and drink through a *bombilla*.

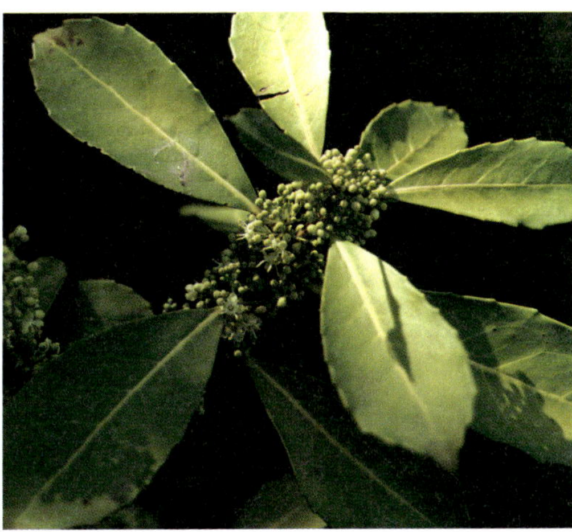

• It can be enjoyed hot in a variety of ways, including in the traditional gourd with a *bombilla* (metal filter straw) or prepared as tea, with the leaves or bags similar to tea bags.

• **Warning.** This drink is not recommended for anxiety, high blood pressure, heart complications, insomnia, gastritis or duodenal ulcers.

ESSENTIAL OILS FROM A TO Z

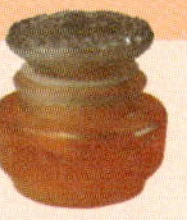

PATCHOULI

This essential's aroma helps to reduce the appetite and increase your energy. It is recommended for use in cellulitis fighting massages, because it helps to reduce water retention. Because of its evoking properties it's recommended to use in a room for meditation. This oil's effects increase if mixed with pine or myrrh.

Safety. In reduced amounts this oil can work as a sedative, in high doses as a stimulant.

ROSE

It has aromatic effects, especially for the physiological and emotional discomforts suffered by women. It acts as a slight anti-depressant, helping to relieve the anxiety caused by weight gain. In a warm bath it can be blended with jasmine and sandalwood to lift up your spirits.

Safety. Do not use during the first four months of pregnancy.

index

Introduction

What are weight problems? 4
Most frequent causes 6
The ideal weight 8
Healthy habits 10
Quality in foods and eating 14
The role of the family 16
Overweight children 18

Diet and Weight Reducing Therapies

Design your own diet 20
A model plan 26
Importance of moving 28
Walking for your health 32
Gym activities 36
Water exercises 38
Reducing pilates 40
Shiatsu against hunger 44
Yoga for weight loss 46

Healing Foods

Essential nutrients 50

Natural Herb Remedies

Natural help 56

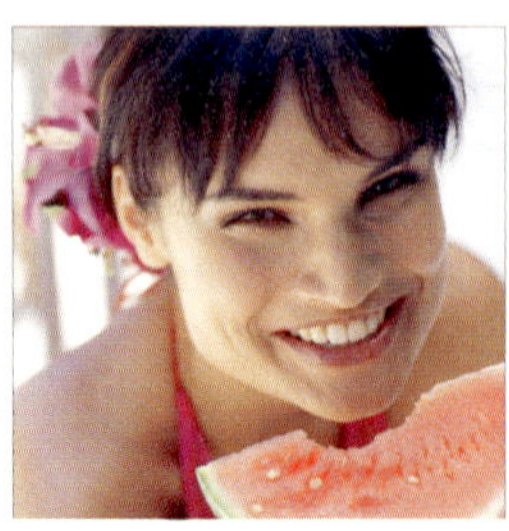